Beyond the darkness of dementia

Finding hope when all appears lost

Wendy Hall

First paperback edition June 2023

Book cover design by Daria DiCieli

Book cover photography by Earthbound Studio

ISBN 978-0-6451185-2-0 (paperback)

www.dementiadoulas.com.au

In dedication to Ian

Thank you for sharing in a vision to make the world of dementia a better place for all those who pass through it. Know that your ongoing dedication to a cause greater than yourself will never be forgotten by those you have inspired along the way.

CONTENTS

Preface

The conversations in this book are ones that many families supporting someone with dementia wish they could have had or should have had. They are conversations that often have nowhere to land, no one to have them with or no one who would fully understand. The content that is shared is, at times raw, but it's also genuine and reflective in its messaging. Many of the words are from those who are walking, or who have previously walked, the path through dementia, and it's their insights that assist us in paving the way forward for a better tomorrow. It's not about getting stuck in blame – 'Someone could have or should have – ', but it does acknowledge the challenges families and support providers face every day with a lack of acknowledgment and suitable, time appropriate resources that never seem to answer all the difficult questions.

This doesn't promise to be an easy read, but it will be an honest one. By addressing issues often faced by families in a sensitive way, I hope they may feel less overwhelmed by what is ultimately to come. It's often fear of the unknown that results in fractured relationships and routines of life, well before the impact of dementia comes into play. When the bigger picture is clearer to see, everyone involved is better placed to tackle issues with a planned rollout that takes each moment one step at a time.

This book was created with family members and support providers in mind. The hope is that it will help in some small way to provide connection and support for those who find themselves trying to navigate and understand the dementia journey. The dialogue contained may also be useful for those living with dementia. It may open up conversations that never appeared to have a starting point or created an uncertainty about what to say or how to say it. May this be a resource for assisting with lost words and meanings or for framing conversations into their intended context.

A theme of letters flows throughout so that topics covered remain relatable and relevant. The words shared come from the hearts and experiences of those who are walking the path or have done so in the past. The messages throughout will hopefully reassure all those impacted by advancing dementia that the future they face isn't one they face alone. The sharing of insights and experiences brings a confirmation that throughout the difficult times there are moments to be treasured while reminding families of the need to take a well-deserved breath, and to do so without the burden of guilt so many often carry.

Through the writing of letters, a vessel for true expression has been created. Families have been able to tap into the dialogue sitting beneath the surface which, for many has lain dormant and hidden over several years. The writing of the letters provided an avenue for families to say what they wanted to say in the way they wanted to say it. The letters provided the words that were often jumbled and disconnected, giving them a place to land.

By family members bravely sharing their experiences, my hope is that, in some small way they will help someone, somewhere, to feel more supported and a little less alone. This book has been able to capture and validate stories that often go unheard, stories which those living them think there's no one in the world who could possibly understand. I hope to give these stories meaning and purpose so others will see the value in their own personal stories and be reassured that by sharing them, they provide an insight into a world that to many remains a mystery. It is hoped that these contributions will flow on more widely and influence the shape of what dementia care will look like in the future.

I hope this book becomes a useful tool for many, with ideas for how to move forward through the dementia trajectory. I hope that it empowers families and support providers not only with a voice but with strategies to stock their personal toolkit. It contains ideas for better connections and for creating opportunities to share in reflections of the past, a time that for many living with dementia becomes a safe and reassuring space.

Dementia should no longer mean life can't go on, but instead highlight the need for a better structure to be put in place framing and providing insights into what the future could look like. It's being honest and real about the likely challenges that will be faced and the need to put supports into position today. Families should no longer be waiting for the storm to hit before they open the 'how to get through it' manual. By better supporting families at the outset, these firsthand insights will assist in shifting care sector preconceptions about what families need to care for and support someone with dementia, and so influence and drive change in a way that will tangibly influence the way dementia care evolves in times to come.

Beyond the darkness of dementia, is a raw and real account of the lived experience of supporting and caring for someone with dementia and we realise it underestimates the power in its messaging. While providing an opportunity for families to share with others the frustrations, challenges, sadness, and despair, it also becomes a place to share the joy, happiness and sense of hope that's so often lost amongst the chaos. By keeping it real, we stand a better chance of preparing families for what's to come on some level, so they are as ready as possible for the moments dementia will ultimately bring.

1 • Understanding the hand that's dealt

'The effects of being a family caregiver, though sometimes positive, are generally negative, with high rates of burden and psychological morbidity as well as social isolation, physical ill-health, and financial hardship.'

- Brodaty & Donkin, 2009, p.217

Imagine ....

Imagine if families and those diagnosed with dementia were better prepared, right from the start, for what was to come so they'd be better informed to decide how things would play out.

As I write this, I do so with clear intention: to help keep family members or support providers at the centre of what's going on around them. If you're supporting someone in their caring role, I hope you'll also find opportunity to take on the messages for yourself. Dementia is an area where those impacted often feel undeserving of any attention or support, feeling that the person with the diagnosis of dementia is the only one in the scenario who can justifiably claim to be 'suffering' or in need of additional support.

But when we offer and provide better support to those that take on a care role, we in turn acknowledge their place in the bigger picture, their needs, and what they might find useful from those of us surrounding them. The flow on effect is a more consistent care approach that better meets the mark for the person with dementia and their families, today and well into the future.

As I reflected on the way I wanted to help families connect with others through a shared experience, I spoke with Angela, who had lost her husband to dementia 11 years ago. I shared with her the importance of writing such a book to ensure families felt heard and listened to. I mentioned my concern of hoping the messaging wasn't too strong or overwhelming.

Angela reassured me that honest and open conversations about how to care for someone with dementia had been missing for her. She spoke openly about the messaging she had previously heard at forums, seen in written publications and within support groups and how confronting and difficult it had been to hear at times.

Angela shared that for her, if the dialogue became too heavy in a specific moment, she would stop reading or simply walk away. She knew the information was important and would return when she felt ready to do so. What Angela highlighted was that she had wanted to be the one to decide the relevance of information provided and not have someone else make the decision about what she should have access to.

This valuable insight helped me see the need for a metaphorical bookmark to ensure there was always the opportunity for the reader to pause and come back to a marked spot when the time was right.

The impact of dementia

Those living within our broader communities often go about their day-to-day lives untouched by dementia at a personal level, but unfortunately as the incidence of dementia continues to grow within our society, that is likely to change over the coming years. While there are over 400,000 people currently living with a diagnosis of dementia in Australia, by 2050, that number is predicted to increase to around 1 million people.

Globally, 55 million people have a diagnosis of dementia and by 2050 this figure too is expected to climb to around 139 million. It is an unfortunate reality that from a statistical perspective many have already been touched by dementia or will be at some point in the future.

Firsthand experience of dementia will likely become a reality with a known diagnosis of either a family member, friend, close contact, or themselves. How prepared are we as a community for the increasing incidence of dementia? Does anyone ever feel truly ready for what lies ahead in this regard? While most of us lack the necessary skills needed to tackle dementia, we must be better prepared heading into the future. For too long, those impacted by advancing dementia, the person themselves, their families, friends and even care staff, have gone it alone, feeling unsupported and lost in an area for which we should be better prepared.

With an aged care system already facing crisis and shortage of sufficient funding around the world, the unfortunate reality is there won't be any quick fixes any time soon. Our best way forward is to become more self-sufficient: looking after our own better, creating new care models for those impacted by dementia, educating our communities in risk reduction measures and how to better support those impacted by dementia we so often walk past in the street.

The non-textbook reality of dementia

Dementia is so many little things all rolled into one that together create the big things we often see. The experience of dementia may be a new world for many or something others have tackled before. Maybe, in hindsight, family members have questioned early signs which lacked any clear meaning at the time. In the earlier stages, dementia may have been seen through the need to write a list or for a gentle reminder. It may have been the finishing of a sentence, or the offering of a forgotten word, the finding of a misplaced name, a familiar face, a lost set of keys or a car in a carpark. The signs were likely there but masked by every day, normal forgetting or by a barrier built so high to minimise those on the outside seeing in.

Dementia can be the moments of confusion noticed in another, the uncharacteristic behaviours and reactions that went unexplained. It can look like confrontations over the smallest of things that historically wouldn't even have been an issue. Now the frustration experienced and expressed over a failed or incomplete task is tangible. It may have been the inability to cope with, or to be productive at work. It may have been in the difficulty with the simplest of tasks, that were once second nature now requiring more effort and concentration. The pot left on the stove top, the scones too long in oven, the fear in one's eyes when scolded, all signal that life is now heading in a direction where it is unlikely to ever remain the same again.

Dementia takes a direct aim at a person's confidence, resulting in a recoil from social opportunities that at one time may have been embraced and enjoyed. It changes relationships leaving them difficult to navigate and understand, with nobody within a family unit sure of how to connect or what role they will now play. Dementia changes a person within a family unit from someone others have always looked to for advice and turns the tables so the person with dementia now relies on the guidance of others. Dementia will redefine what a family unit looks like and the roles everyone must now step into.

The biggest impact I have witnessed for someone newly diagnosed with dementia is the impact on their lifestyle and personhood. Someone with an early diagnosis of dementia can be experiencing a few issues with their memory and thought processes, but still be working in paid employment, running family budgets and households. Yet, overnight, with a diagnosis of dementia, the impact on a person's confidence and self-esteem can leave them feeling as if they no longer have anything to contribute well before their actual abilities have been lost by dementia.

Dementia will make it difficult for someone to balance the weight of their own expectations of self with the expectation of others. This can result in continued blows to self-esteem from repeated correcting by others, reminding of repeated words or questions, leaving the person with dementia feeling they are now thought of as stupid or incompetent. Dementia creates a dependency on others for the simplest things in life, from finding the coffee cups, to putting away the milk.

It's a long-drawn-out diagnosis that goes on and on with frequent losses, often without answers but new waves of emotion to navigate. A diagnosis of dementia can cause mixed feelings from relief about having an answer for why things are changing, to devastation and sadness for a vibrant life now continuing to be lost and not knowing who to turn to when so many people are talking with words that fall away, and having to navigate the shock, anger and fear that remains.

Searching for a starting line

An ongoing struggle for families is not knowing what to do, when to do what needs to be done and where to turn for help when it's needed. They often lack a starting point because dementia rarely offers one. Families usually find themselves coming in at different points of the disease trajectory and are often unsure whether the actions they put in motion to support their family member with dementia are overcompensating, undercompensating, or truly hitting the intended mark.

Families often comment that they're not really sure which path is the right one for them during the earlier stages of dementia, a time where things don't make sense, a time where families often take a step back, trying to get away from the confusion and the chaos. The earlier stages of the disease can leave families feeling tired and overwhelmed by the guilt as they try to navigate their own feelings of helplessness.

As dementia progresses, families must somehow learn to adapt to the changes experienced by the person with dementia on many different levels. There will likely be further impairment of memory and increased confusion continuing to cloud the ability to orientate oneself to new or familiar surroundings.

Voices that no longer have meaning or familiarity can lead to strong feelings of disconnection. There are memories of a home that is missed but never forgotten, feelings of abandonment and being discarded as strangers appear, pretending to be people from the past, impostors.

The person with dementia can feel like an outcast, existing in a parallel universe while looking into another world, all the while not feeling included, or connected in any way.

Family members should also keep in mind that dementia is a slow decline over months to years, not hours to days. If sudden changes do occur, we're likely looking at something totally different going on for the person and a further assessment is warranted from their General Practitioner (GP) to rule out something treatable like a urinary tract infection, delirium, pain, or other conditions.

Vince's story …

During my paramedic days I was tasked to, 'an older man, who was very unwell'. On arrival at his home, it appeared as if there was no one home. We slowly entered the house through the unlocked front door to find a man semi-naked, lying on the lounge room floor and mumbling. My first thoughts were that he had quite advanced dementia. We were unable to connect with him through conversation or understand what he was trying to say.

Shortly after, Vince's son arrived and shared that his father didn't have dementia and he'd never seen him in this state before. Nothing obvious was showing up for us, but upon arrival at hospital, an assessment uncovered a severe urinary tract infection from which Vince was not doing well. Following treatment, Vince was lucky to fully recover and resume life as he'd previously known.

This story highlights the need for a thorough assessment when changes to memory, thought processes or other unusual changes occur to ensure treatable conditions aren't missed through assumptions being made.

Credit where credit is due

Dementia gets blamed for so much, for fractures in families, destroying lives, being a burden on the health system, but in many cases, we, as support providers, often give up on the person well before dementia has even started to have a debilitating effect on them. We give dementia too much credit for how it affects individuals and families and therefore, early on, give away the ability to put dementia in its place, and the differences we can make.

Dementia does certainly have an impact on everyday life, making normal everyday struggles and challenges more difficult. However, support providers and family members can bring even the smallest amount of normality back where all appears lost. It's never easy, but with the right supports in place it can sometimes be a little easier than before. Knowing where we, as individuals, fit in all of this is so important, the role we can play, have capacity to play and essentially, the role we might want to play.

We need to somehow reframe our thinking about dementia, to see it for what it is, a debilitating brain disease that makes everyday life harder. Because we can't see the damage that's occurring, it means we can find it harder to connect with the person. When we argue with a person with dementia, when we correct them and remind them, we're actually going up against dementia, the debilitating brain disease. The odds are stacked in dementia's favour, and it will always win. It's not the person themselves, but the disease that is unrelenting and unwilling to compromise.

Dementia takes away the person's ability to reason and it's an emotionally charged response and reaction that we will often see. If there's shouting and anger, it only fuels the fire and the person with dementia will ultimately feel under some sort of attack. And when any of us are placed in this position and feel like that, we're all likely to come out swinging. Things may seem impossible and unachievable, overwhelming, but by taking each day as it comes and having a plan in place, working on things bit-by-bit, then true progress can be made, and new ways discovered for relating to the person with dementia on a more personal level.

'We don't even know after 5 years what type of dementia Dad even has.'

- Daughter of dad with dementia –

Ensuring families feel heard

Dear Dementia,

You are an insidious terminal disease that has no cure. You slowly take away everything from a person, while loved ones, family, friends, acquaintances etc., just have to stand by and watch this happen, whilst feeling so heartbroken and helpless. We slowly say goodbye to the person we love, while they are still there. You are so very, very cruel.

There are no words to describe it.

From a caring wife - Jenny

After encouraging family members to share their thoughts through the writing of a letter, I wanted to try it for myself. I wrote the following to 'family members', as I sought to express my sadness and remorse for a failing system so many find themselves in. I did so in the hope that by starting with an apology, we, as a system, may find ourselves better positioned for real change.

I share my disappointment in a system filled with caring and well-meaning individuals, all who have a passion and drive for making a difference but are so often not supported in their practice to do so. This letter is, I hope, a starting point for moving forward, to acknowledge where we, as a system, have inadvertently let families down. As a system, we need to look towards a brighter future where we take ownership and responsibility for the roles we play, knowing there are so many opportunities to do things differently. A new day is dawning where we can meet the needs of families in ways previously not thought possible and take the next steps together.

Dear Family Member,

I write this to you with a feeling of angst and sadness for how much we, as a society, system and sector have let you down. We've let you down, not once, not twice but from the moment you got on this crazy ride called dementia. We waited for you, until the world crumbled around you. We waited for you, knowing you were coming and that a crisis would turn your world upside down and inevitably send you in our direction.

That crisis may present in the form of a simple fall in the shower, getting lost returning from the shops, meals in the fridge left uneaten, a long-awaited holiday cut short because of the confusion and chaos that ensued. Or it may have been following hospital visits where things were never the same again after dementia made itself known. We knew these times were coming and we waited, with forms at the ready, pens poised. Those moments did come, and although you had little to no warning, and you were taken by shock and surprise, we were there at the ready.

Your world collapsed in a way you could never have imagined. You felt helpless and didn't know where to turn. So, in your hour of need, you were pointed in our direction. We, as a sector, as a system, were there ready and waiting for you. We had trained and developed systems for this moment in time. And it was then that we opened our doors, and we didn't invite you in, we ushered you in. It was a busy day, and we had many more people to see, all of them just like you. But we told you we were ready.

Instead of taking your hand, we handed you a pen and a heap of forms to fill out. All to be done in your time of overwhelming confusion. Instead of that cup of tea or stiff drink you so desperately needed, we told you to take a seat or join a six-month waiting list. When time stood still for you, and you weren't sure which way was up and which way was down, we told you to wait. But we were supposed to be ready for you.

We looked into your teary eyes, full of shock and despair, and instead of guidance and hope, we said, 'I'm sorry, there's nothing we can do. The limited treatment available will neither fix, nor cure, but you could join a drug trial.' We extinguished that small flame, that small flicker of light, a chance of hope, without a second thought. Dementia, that's just the way it is. Do we care? You bet we care. But we just don't know what to do with a disease with no cure, no alleged positive outcomes. So, we did the only thing we knew to do. We went all process on you. We defaulted to our clinical comfort zone, that place where we're trained to fix and provide a remedy. At the time you sought direction, we offered you not a hand to hold but a handful of helpful brochures, handfuls of assurances that we would sort everything out. We said we would provide you with services, offer respite and maybe even a small financial allowance. At that moment, where you wanted direction, instead of slowing things down for you, we accidently sped everything up. Instead of empowering you to tackle this disease, we disempowered you by putting your future in the hands of others.

So, you went home, and you cried. You cried because nobody got it. No one understood. And no one seemed to truly care. You put away the brochures thinking you would look at them when things settled a little. You thought it was all too hard and you would find a way to deal with it on your own. You knew it wouldn't be perfect, but you knew what you had to do to just keep things ticking over. You retreated into a world where no one could connect with you: a world so far removed from the one you'd known. Who would you now talk to? Who could possibly understand?

Friends began retreating, afraid of not knowing what to say or how to connect. Family tried their best and it was only the family dog that seemed to have a knowing look in his eyes. This would be your new world; this world you would make for yourself, a world where outsiders could try to infiltrate with our great ideas and our version of understanding. We said we were ready for you.

You quietly soldiered on for another 10 years, living a life of uncertainty. Day by day you put one foot in front of the other. You smiled politely to others. You told us you were ok. You couldn't risk another lecture on what you should be doing or when and how you should be doing it. Often, we would say, 'There's a website you could check out, full of links you could follow!', but we forgot to even ask if you had or knew how to use a computer. And then, after years of juggling life, your world crashed down in a way that you could never have imagined. You weren't ready for this. But we were ready for this, and we knew you would one day be back. The craziness from all those years ago started all over again.

More decisions needed to be made immediately, with heightened emotions, a lack of understanding and support. More brochures appeared. Higher care was strongly advised as the next option with more decisions to be made. You looked to the left and then to the right. There was no one by your side, but you felt something from behind.

You were being pushed into a direction you weren't ready or prepared for. You were on a moving walkway that was only going in one direction. You weren't ready for this and lacked understanding of where it was taking you. But we were, we are waiting for you. And like driving a car, we turn off the engine and take the keys off you and tell you we'll take it from here.

Kindest regards, 'The Aged Care Sector'

Melissa and Tim's story is one that is all too common: a married couple with adult children experience first-hand the devastation of a partner being diagnosed with younger onset dementia.

We'll share in their story over the coming chapters to highlight the different touchpoints throughout their experience of dementia where there wasn't anyone waiting for them to guide them in a way where they maintained control. So, as a family, they were forced to navigate the dementia path on their own. We share in the learnings from their story to ensure others don't go it alone in the future.

Melissa's story …

Melissa was a 54-year-old primary school teacher and her husband Tim, was 52 years old, working as an accountant, when he was diagnosed with frontotemporal lobar degeneration (FTLD), a progressive, neurologic type of dementia that primarily damages the frontal and temporal lobes of the brain.

The onset of FTLD often occurs earlier than in Alzheimer's disease and someone diagnosed with FTLD will frequently exhibit impaired social abilities and marked disinhibitions. As the behavioural aspects of Tim's disease worsened, the care and support his family were now able to provide became increasingly complicated. Melissa was finding it more and more difficult to connect with Tim and to just sit and have conversations like they used to.

This was a couple who had been in professional roles with good incomes. They were goal orientated, committed to each other, and were busying themselves creating the life they had dreamed of. Forgetfulness and unusual behaviours were noted early. Confusion was increasing for Tim and work becoming more draining on him. Explanations for these changes were a series of guesswork by his family and limited connection with his general practitioner (GP). This pre-diagnostic time for Tim and his family put all of them in a holding pattern as they attempted to make sense of life without an actual diagnosis. The thought of dementia was not a consideration due to Tim's age. It was thought likely he was experiencing depression or another debilitating condition.

Confrontations within the family started to arise as Tim's behaviours continued to flag concern. The time came for frank conversations with Tim's GP and eventually medical advice was sort. After an extended and slow process, a diagnosis was eventually given. The whole family were in shock and disbelief as they tried to grapple with the enormity of the diagnosis they now faced. Melissa tried her best to take on both roles of their partnership while trying to maintain her role as a teacher.

The loss of Tim's job earlier than anticipated would herald the bigger losses of hopes, plans and dreams of what their retirement years should have looked like. Melissa spent many hours researching Tim's condition and even considered getting a second opinion as she grappled with the future she now faced as Tim's primary support provider. Tim's disinhibited behaviours escalated, and his care needs continued to rise.

Continuing in her role as a teacher, a job she'd done her entire working life, and one she enjoyed and which provided purpose and meaning for Melissa, was no longer possible. Melissa was not only dealing with the loss and grief over her own identity and career, but also finding herself dealing with the rest of the family's grief and loss as well.

Her adult children began to distance themselves and Melissa found she was constantly trying to bridge this gap as well. Friends she relied on over many years were suddenly absent, and neighbours were now excluding her from their community gatherings. The stigma surrounding Tim's behaviours was more and more prominent and isolation began to set in.

Even during these early years, the issues that began to surface for Tim and Melissa, and the complexities that developed due to a diagnosis of dementia, are often down played or unacknowledged in any form. This is the point where families and their support networks need to be better prepared for what is to come, to take away the associated fears and provide opportunity for formulating their own plan for how they will move forward as a family and a united front.

Preparing for a better tomorrow …

What could you do to better understand what dementia is ……?

Family perspective …

'There had been many conversations and decisions that seemed to come so very quickly once Dad was diagnosed with Alzheimer's. And the saying that 'you don't know what you don't know' couldn't have been truer at that time.'

-Daughter of dad with dementia-

Just remember that …

Dementia creates a world so far removed from the one any of us have ever known, one that's missing an instruction manual, and no one truly understands.

-Wendy Hall-

2 • The reality of the day to day

'Memory is a salient aspect of identity. The loss of personal memories can be challenging for persons experiencing cognitive problems and for their spouses, since shared memories often constitute partners' sense of togetherness.'

- Hernandez et al., 2019 p.1166

Imagine ....

Imagine if families could look forward to today rather than living with the dread of an unknown tomorrow.

For many families and partners, the day to day of caring for someone with dementia in their home environment is done on their own. Yet family members show up not because they want to sign up for such a full-on workload, but because of a commitment they made to a mother, father, partner, child, neighbour, through a sense of duty or just because they care about another human being and don't believe anyone could come close to caring like they do.

Families continue to find themselves caring and 'winging it' until a turning point happens, usually in the form of some sort of crisis - a fall, a trip away, a hospital visit, an event that turns their lives upside down and changes their lives.

Their hands are forced, and they're directed to the system that will take over from here. Someone else will handle it and they don't have to worry anymore. But families do worry. They don't stop worrying. In many cases, they worry more because they're no longer able to assist the person like they used to. They've lost their sense of purpose and feel totally disconnected from the person as well as life around them.

They visit their loved one in care as though they're visiting an unwell patient in hospital. The interesting part is, their loved one often isn't unwell, it's just that their care needs have increased. So rather than a meaningful connection being established, family members often sit in silence or partake in generalised conversations just to pass the time.

Over the years, it's usually during this stage that a family member will likely come to me and say they think they might be developing dementia too. Whilst statistically, that may be the case, I ask them to think about the role they now play.

They support and provide care to their family member with dementia 24 hours a day, 7 days a week, over 365 days of the year and wonder why their memory is failing them and they're feeling confused at times. They're exhausted. The interesting comparison is we wouldn't put care or nursing staff through those same hours. Why? Because they'd burn out.

Melissa's story (continued) …

Tim and Melissa's children became estranged from both their father and their mother. Melissa was now forced to try to get through each day within an isolated bubble that had now formed around them both. As Tim's needs continued to rise and his behaviours continuing to escalate, Melissa made the heart-breaking decision to put Tim into care. Melissa now carried the burden on her own, feeling like she'd betrayed Tim, feeling exhausted but with little to no support around her. Her own health was becoming compromised, her energy levels depleted, and she could no longer maintain the pace she had once set.

Melissa tried to rebuild ties with family and friends that had severed over time. There was some success, but she felt through her grief that many connections from the past were now lost to her. While Tim resided in higher care, Melissa was still consumed with visiting him and trying to ensure he had the things he needed and enjoyed. Melissa felt that while the 24hr care she had provided to Tim in their home had ceased, the weight of caring hadn't changed significantly for her: the difference being she was now not considered a carer even though it was the role she still clearly identified with.

Weeks turned into months and Tim's decline became more evident: the cognitive changes Melissa had known were then now added to by the significant changes to Tim's mobility. Tim was eventually considered to be at the end-of-life stage. Melissa felt shattered and broken but stayed with Tim throughout his last days. Following Tim's death, Melissa's emotions were again continuing into a new phase of grief at the loss of her husband, life partner and the guilt that she 'should' have done things differently, or 'better', that in some way she had let Tim down. Following Tim's death, Melissa's busyness ramped up. She had a funeral to organise and financial affairs to attend to.

She did this while trying to help others with their grief and remorse. Life slowly restarted and over time Melissa was then able to start rebuilding her new 'self'. While she would never truly get over the loss of Tim, her friends, dreams and identity, Melissa did start rebuilding a new version of herself over the coming years. She changed in ways she could never have imagined.

Changes happening right from the start

No one will ever offer care like those who know and love the person with dementia most. But it will always come at a cost. The stakes are always high. Partners and family are often juggling their own health concerns, their own families. They give and give until something breaks. Chaos ensues and their family member ends up in the closest bed available, not necessarily one the person or family would have chosen for themselves.

We need to think about the experience of visiting a relative or friend in hospital. Reflect for a moment on what it does to us. We often find ourselves acting and speaking differently, maybe quieter, and more constrained. If we feel comfortable in doing so, we may ask the doctors and nurses what is happening. We don't usually attempt to assert ourselves and try to take on a role within the environment that isn't on offer to us. It's likely we would change how we act considerably compared to within our own homes. Likewise, someone with dementia also loses the cues they're accustomed to, especially if the cues were coming from others around them which can cause confusion for them.

Given we're conditioned to play a passive role within a hospital setting and given a care home environment is a replication of this, it's no surprise family and friends will act differently here too. It's common to take a back seat, hoping someone will update them, hoping their loved one is receiving the best care from the best staff possible, feeling helpless that there's nothing they can do to contribute.

The following is in tribute to ...

In loving memory of Kym, from Jenie, Amy & Matthew

Dear Dementia,

I saw you hovering at our door, unsure of who you were or what your business was. You were a creepy shadow outside, until you showed your face & decided to move in full time. At first, we were scared, we didn't like you at all. You changed my husband, I had to watch you with frustration & anger take over my husband's world. My children had to watch their dad become someone they didn't recognise through frustration & denial. You barged your way into our home uninvited. Like a bad smell from a garbage bin, you were always there.

We wanted you to leave 'get out of our home', our safe place, that brought us so much joy, but you stayed, and you were persistent. We were exhausted trying to fight you, you are strong and relentless, you are ruthless, and you bring so much sadness. We were fighting a losing battle, our armour was scratched and dented from fighting you. Every day we fought while you got stronger, we became weak.

Then one day, our family decided we were not going to let you win. We changed the way we saw you; we upped the game plan; we knew you weren't leaving... you were here to stay. We had to change the way we fought you so we could survive this time you spent with us. We decided we weren't going to be frightened anymore. We weren't going to let you bring that negativity to our happy family. We stood as a united front. We swapped anger for quality time. We chose to use our energy on things that brought us unforgettable memories. We made the most of every day. We laughed, and we cried happy tears whenever we could.

We experienced joy with you. We no longer saw you as a burden but a member of our family that came to stay. We made the most of having you around. We adjusted to your being. We didn't know how long you were coming to stay.

You no longer live with us; you moved out permanently. We had to say goodbye. It was sad and heart-breaking when you left because you had to take my husband with you, the man our family loved so dearly. We now look back at you with fond memories.

We met so many wonderful people when you came to live with us. We taught ourselves to love you, not because we wanted to…. but because we had to. We couldn't live life hating you…, that is not living, that is existing. My husband deserved more.

I see you hovering at other people's doors now and making your way into their lives. I hope they learn to accept you as our family did. I hope they get the quality time and special happy moments that we did. I hope they learn to live with you as we did.

Dear Dementia…… we miss you.

From Jenie

Through the eyes of another

Before we search for answers as to how we can better support someone living with dementia, we must first take time to understand life from their perspective. This isn't at all easy and most of us have no parallel experience from our own life experiences to align with what it might be like, unless perhaps someone has experienced an amnesic episode. Meet Roger.

Roger's story …

I remember back to my earlier days in a dementia support role working with Roger. Roger had a diagnosis of Alzheimer's disease and lived with his wife within the family home. He would always turn up to any event or gathering looking sad and disconnected. He had no interest in participating in discussions or finding a way forward. Roger would show up in support of his wife, and he'd just go through the motions.

One day I had an opportunity to chat with Roger and asked him how he was getting on. I enquired as to whether he was interested in participating in an upcoming event. His reply was, 'What's the point?'. I asked him what he meant by this and felt saddened by his reply, 'I hate going anywhere and doing anything. I'm embarrassed that I can't even remember a friend's name, and everyone keeps telling me I'm repeating myself. It's easier to just not go out at all'.

This was a precious insight into Roger's world and what life was like for him. I treasure this lesson to this day. Roger taught me to ensure I never second guess what it might be like to live with dementia. Unless it comes from someone with dementia directly, I will always take feedback as hearsay. Roger helped me reframe my thoughts and the questions I asked. I would move forward not telling someone with dementia where they needed to head but instead asking what it was that they needed from me? How could I do better in this space?

Roger needed me to support his independence by giving him back a sense of self-worth, to do what I could to make him feel as comfortable as I could to restore the confidence he'd lost. What I realised was that Roger didn't need me to speak or tell him more. What he needed from me was my own self-awareness for how I conducted myself around him, how I spoke, the words I used, how I included him and how I set him up for success, and not to leave him feeling uncomfortable or disconnected.

Dementia can leave someone feeling angry, frustrated, and saddened due to the grieving they experience for all they were able to once do.

The answers aren't always easy to find, but sometimes the answers come from the questions yet to be asked.

-Wendy Hall-

Navigating the world of dementia without a map

Families are often unsure how the aged care system works. Like characters in a movie, no one knows the story line or where it's all heading. Those working within the aged care sector are likely to know how the story will unfold, and moving forward we must get better at taking families along for the ride and no longer leave them standing on the outside looking in. As families continue trying to navigate the aged care system at every stage of the dementia trajectory, more can be done to prepare for them to play a more prominent role in care provision while feeling that their voices are being heard.

Over the years I've often questioned why we weren't educating families earlier about what was to come so we could in effect hand them back the reins for supporting their loved one. With an aged care sector experiencing shortages of funding and resources, families empowered to plan for tomorrow and for what is to come have the potential to become a well needed resource in an already overwhelmed system. Families would not only be better placed in their understanding of where they are headed but may also be a driving force in informing aged care leaders of more productive and efficient ways forward.

'I don't want to be trying to sort everything out, I just want to be the daughter.'

- Daughter of dad with dementia –

Bronwyn's story ...

Bronwyn attended a family session I was conducting and became emotional as she shared her experience of visits with her mother in a high care environment. Bronwyn described the heartache she felt and the feelings of being dismissed and rejected each time she entered her mother's room. She would regularly feel an immense pain knowing her mother didn't want to connect with her as she would raise her hand indicating she wanted her to stop talking before she'd even had a chance to finish her sentence.

What hurt Bronwyn even more was how happy and comfortable her mother appeared to be when Bronwyn's teenage daughter would enter the room. Her mother's face would light up in response and she could only watch from the sidelines how much joy her daughter's visits brought. Bronwyn was confused and devastated that she had, somewhere along the line, lost that same connection she'd once had too. She couldn't understand why she felt the way she did and why her own mother would respond in such a way that hurt her.

We took a moment to reflect on the visit she was experiencing with her mother and to try to see the world through her mother's eyes. There were two aspects we discussed that provided a perspective Bronwyn had not considered. The first was how we, as adults, have been conditioned to interact with others. While being well-meaning, we often ask open-ended questions to express our interest in the lives of others. How are you? What have you been up to today? What did you have for lunch? We do so in the hope that the other person will open up and share their experiences of what's happening in their world with us.

For someone living with dementia, this line of questioning can often represent a threat. Questions might need a response they may get right or wrong. If they get the answer wrong, there's often an awareness they'll be corrected. This can bring about feelings of failure or inadequacy. For someone living with dementia, these questions often leave them feeling tested.

If we ask someone with dementia if they've had any visitors and they respond with, 'Tony came to see me the other day', we may be quick to respond with, 'He can't have visited you, he's still living in London.' It's an instant failure and likely to shut down any further interactions. This response may have resulted from Tony's name being mentioned, seeing a photo of Tony or maybe there'd been a call with Tony on the phone. Whatever the reason, the emotional memory will remind the person that answering questions will always come with an element of risk.

We explored further how (to stereotype) a teenager visit may unfold. I asked Bronwyn how her daughter's visit would play out, and she reflected that she'd share with her grandmother what she'd been up to and what she'd been doing with her friends. And there we had it. No questions. Her daughter simply took on the role of storyteller and all Grandma had to do was listen. She could sit back and enjoy the sound of her granddaughter's voice, her facial expressions and the smiles. She could even throw in the occasional, 'Hmmm, ahhh', just to show she was staying connected.

Grandma was likely to be lost in the conversation and not understanding or following the chain of events, but that's unlikely to be what was important to her. What was important was the connection she felt and the energy her granddaughter brought to every visit.

The second aspect we explored was the nature of Alzheimer's disease, the diagnosis Bronwyn's mum had. We needed to recall the experience as one where the person is effectively going back in time with their memories. It's useful to think of the memory like a filing cabinet, which is empty when we're born. As we continue through life, we fill up our memory filing cabinet with skills, knowledge, and wisdom collected along the way.

What Alzheimer's disease does is to rip out the front or most recent files first, so the person is effectively going back in time. That's why someone may not remember their son visited this morning but clearly recounts the fishing trip they went on with their grandfather when they were fifteen years old. Those older memories are tucked safely right at the back of the memory filing cabinet.

What this may also mean is by going back in time, Bronwyn's mum may have thought she was younger than she actually was.

Instead of thinking she was 85 years old, she may have thought she was more around 40 years old. You then start to see the confusion this can create. It wouldn't equate for her to think Bronwyn was her daughter. She would more likely be thinking her granddaughter was her daughter. If her granddaughter was similar in appearance to how Bronwyn had been at a similar age, you can better appreciate Grandma's perspective in all of this.

We tried to reframe why Bronwyn's daughter was possibly having more success at visiting in the hope that she could think of a different approach to try herself in moving forward. This will always be easier said than done, but bringing perspective to a situation at least assists someone like Bronwyn to be open about the hurt they're feeling while knowing it's a person's dementia that pushes others away and not the person they remain at the core. Looking at different ways to connect is where we'll head in future chapters.

Dementia Prayer – By Robyn
(Written for her husband's experience with dementia)

With time our memories dim and fade, it's the course of life that we accept. Whilst living with dementia as such, we sadly look at this with regret. Our younger years how vivid in mind, my yesterdays not nearly as kind. Be patient with me as I've lost my way, remember better times and for me please pray, that one day this pain of loss will be gone, together forever and forever beyond …

What gets left behind?

We often focus so much on what dementia takes away that we forget to look at what it leaves behind. When we pivot and readjust where we're looking for hope, opportunities present themselves in ways that help clear what appears to be overgrown paths heading off into the unknown.

Dementia can't:

- touch a strong united family unit.

- take away the person who remains hidden behind the wall of dementia.

- silence the voices of families.

- change our ability to still meet the person's needs.

- lessen the importance of surrounding the person with a community of care.

- change the need to create environments offering a sense of peace and calm to support the person with dementia and their family to get through each day.

Where to head next?

The system must get better at reducing the surprises on a trajectory that has so much certainty about it. By developing the Dementia Doula role, we at Dementia Doulas International became committed to bridging this gap in a way not seen before.

This new role ensures families feel better supported throughout the entire dementia trajectory, making room for honest conversations with families at a time when they are ready to have them. These conversations can be had in a way that takes everyone along for the ride, and with someone they know they can trust.

I will continue to reference the role of the Dementia Doula throughout this book so you, in your role of family member or other support provider, are given an insight into the future we see for dementia care and the impact we believe we can all have when we come together for a common cause with a similar passion.

Families need permission to keep living and to do so in a way that supports their own well-being and connectedness with others. Dementia Doulas assist families to live without guilt and needing to self-sacrifice their own needs in order to provide the best care, often to the detriment of their own quality of life.

As we move forward, we begin looking at how families can find their own space for navigating the feelings and emotions living with dementia can bring, to develop and have a solid plan in place to default to when the need arises that leaves them feeling like they're enough, knowing their contributions make a tangible difference to the life of the person with dementia who they care so much about.

But before we launch into well-meaning strategies, we, as an aged care sector must acknowledge that the starting point will always be to earn the trust of families, allowing them a sense of control and enablement, to bring their own people to the table so that support is ongoing, to have everyone on the same page, with a similar agenda.

We need to recognise the contributions of everyone involved, knowing and appreciating that no one gets an easy ride with dementia, but appreciating that together, we can make a difference in this space.

Preparing for a better tomorrow …

What could you do to help those around you understand this better ……?

Family perspective ...

'I don't want others to think I just gave up on him.'

-Wife of husband with dementia-

Just remember that ...

We can no longer leave families in a situation where they're just left at the mercy of a disease that has no right to be calling all the shots.

-Wendy Hall-

3 • Carrying the weight of dementia

'Caregivers for family members with dementia experience depression, anxiety, and stress and also feelings of resentment, helplessness, and hopelessness, in addition to feeling that they have little free time.'

- Day & Anderson, 2011, p. 1

Imagine ...

Imagine a time when the weight families are expected to carry on their own is lightened by those who are best placed to share the load.

Disclaimer: This chapter explores grief and loss in the hope of highlighting how missed or unacknowledged both areas are within dementia care for families and the person with dementia themselves. It is not intended that anyone reading this will attempt to self-diagnose themselves or take on a burden that isn't theirs to carry. What it is intended to do is highlight the different ways we, as individuals, respond and react to stresses or pressures placed upon us at any time throughout our lives; to bring to the fore how we all go through the experience of grief and loss in different ways, with no two experiences being the same. As we explore the different ways and reasons why someone may grieve, it's important to consider now and into the future whether a conversation with a health professional could be of further assistance to you or your loved one.

Understanding grief and loss

Grief can be referred to as a natural response to some type of change or loss. It may be through the death of a loved one but could also be the loss of a home, a lifestyle, the breakdown of a relationship or significant change in health status. Grief is expressed in many ways and can affect every part of someone's life. Grief can impact on emotions, thoughts, behaviours, beliefs, physical health, sense of self and identity, and relationships with others.

The way we feel and think will often affect how we interact with our family and friends. These feelings may leave someone feeling comforted being in the presence of company while others may prefer solitude and to be left alone. There is no set pattern with grief, and while stages of grief may be referred to, everyone will experience grief differently with cultural and circumstantial factors affecting how someone will express and cope with it.

Grief and loss often manifest in ways that are never imagined and hard to identify. This is an area commonly trademarked as being something a person goes through following the death of a loved one. Whilst this is true, dementia sees a variety of losses which lead to grief.

Families often feel alone as they try to navigate the new path that dementia places before them and can feel lost as they seek emotionally safe spaces for sharing what may feel like self-indulgent moments, or where feelings of guilt can be shared and validated.

Families need to find a space where feelings of anger, frustration, and sadness can find a soft place to land. Emotional and physical safety allows families a place to offload their feelings and emotions without fear of being judged or where others may hastily attempt a band aid fix. Without these opportunities, families find themselves constantly treading water without the opportunity to enjoy the view along the way.

Gerry's story ...

I think back to a conversation with Gerry's family many years ago. I had asked his wife and daughter how things had been going over the previous couple of months and they despondently replied with, 'Yes, everything's been okay.' I asked if something specific had happened and they recounted a weekend when Gerry had turned 80 years old, and they'd planned a day to the country and a helicopter flight.

I felt slightly nervous about where the story was heading but knew there had not been any mid-air incidents in the media over the last few weeks. They shared how wonderfully the day had gone and how happy Gerry had been as everything unfolded. Gerry had enjoyed every moment of the experience his family had organised to celebrate his milestone birthday.

The part that brought down the tone of the conversation was related to the drive back home. Gerry's wife shared that everyone was so happy in the car; there was a feeling that they had Gerry back for a moment and they were once again a family.

As the drive continued, Gerry's daughter said, 'Dad, wasn't the helicopter great?'. To which Gerry replied, 'What helicopter?'. The family was shattered. It was as if they'd lost Gerry all over again and expressed sadness that the whole day had been a waste of time and money. Gerry forgetting so quickly meant dementia, for them, had only taken a quick break and had returned way too soon.

We talked about what had happened and I asked Gerry's wife and daughter how he appeared to be feeling on the drive back. His daughter replied, 'Oh, he was happy as anything. He was enjoying the car ride and didn't seem to have a care in the world.' And that was the moment I needed to bring them back to. Gerry was happy and still enjoying the day because of the adventures he'd been on.

I wanted Gerry's family to know that while he had forgotten what had made him happy, his emotional memory ensured his feelings of happiness continued for the next few hours. The good thing for Gerry was that he was still able to recognise himself in photos doing activities that he'd otherwise forgotten. Photos of himself participating in anything brought back a joy he couldn't remember for himself first hand and that was what I encouraged his family to connect with.

This is an example of moments that can really matter for families but often need to be highlighted for them as they're at risk of being covered up by the perceived losses that keep on coming. Those supporting someone with dementia, living with a diagnosis of dementia or working within the dementia care sector, need to practise self-care and be kind to themselves.

What is faced and lived with every day is a shared experience and not one where families should be going it alone. By speaking openly about grief and loss associated with dementia, we become better placed to support everyone affected through what is a difficult and challenging time.

Travelling through grief and loss

Many family members don't identify that what they're feeling could be defined as grief and loss, or that they may be stuck in a state of grief or bereavement. Grief in the context of dementia often spans a long period of time and can be unrelenting.

A myriad of emotions experienced throughout every waking moment of every day and night brings with it a sadness for what has been lost that never leaves or goes away. No one can possibly understand the slow painful decline unless they've experienced it first-hand for themselves.

The experience of grief and loss is unique for everyone going through it. The challenges will differ, and the overwhelming wave of emotions will leave many wondering if the sadness ever ends. The difficulties with a diagnosis of dementia are unrelenting in nature bringing disruption to the lives of those impacted by it. And while there may not be an end point in sight for getting through the experience, which causes the upheaval to life as families know it, it remains important to recognise this time for what it is and have a plan in place for navigating life moving forward.

It's difficult to navigate a time where the starting point is difficult to distinguish and with no idea where it's all supposed to finish. One can feel conflicted, wanting the person back, but not to the life and the hand they've been dealt.

It's challenging to navigate the incomprehensible. The loss of a person through death is such a finite and distinguishable moment in time, but in the case of dementia, this period may span not weeks and months, but more likely many years.

Things for families to consider

Dementia Doulas encourage family members to never be afraid to ask for help. Going it alone and trying to balance all aspects of life won't be easy and won't come with any rewards. Providing insights into what they're feeling with trusted family and friends may not fix what they're going through but may ease the burden and share the weight they carry, reassuring others that listening is often what's needed rather than solutions. Exploring local carer support groups can often bring families into contact with others who understand exactly what they're going through without words even needing to be spoken.

Families need to look after both their physical and emotional health. Dementia is a long road and families deserve to not only build up a resilience for what's to come but also ensure their needs are met along the way. They should ensure they manage stressors that will likely be encountered and seek assistance from a health professional if the challenges faced appear to be taking over.

From a wife who lost her husband to dementia

Dear Alan,

The journey was arduous, the pain is never ending, the regrets are few but still there. I often ask myself, 'What could I have done differently? What could I have done better?' The pain of those two questions will haunt me until the end of time. This wasn't to be our journey; it should have been the adventure we had dreamed about. We were young and looked forward to growing old together.

Instead, we were dealt the blow of this hideous disease. Younger onset dementia robbed us of our future, took your life and burdened me with lifelong memories. Memories that even with time will never be erased.

Regards, Robyn

P.S. My advice to those who will walk in our shoes is this:

NEVER take life for granted,
NEVER assume you have a tomorrow or that your tomorrows were as you dreamed,
NEVER be afraid to reach out for help and support,
And NEVER assume you are qualified for this role.

Remember we weren't trained to take on this huge task, but we strived and continued to strive to do our best. In conclusion, be kind to yourself and those around you, for none of us know what others are dealing with.

Symptoms of Grief

The symptoms of grief may manifest and present themselves in a physical, social, or spiritual way. Common symptoms can include:

- Crying
- Headaches
- Difficulty with sleeping
- Questioning life purpose
- Questioning spiritual beliefs
- Feeling detached

- Isolation from friends and family
- Out of character behaviour
- Worry or anxiety
- Frustration
- Guilt
- Fatigue
- Anger
- Loss of appetite
- Aches and pains
- Stress

Someone living or caring for someone with dementia may find that what they experience is an expression of grief. This type of grief may also be referred to as 'anticipatory grief' as families are often impacted by the anticipation of what lies ahead for them and their family member with dementia, and how they will cope as the challenges continue to increase.

Expressions of grief that families may experience are:

- Feeling tearful but not sure why
- Stressed and overtired
- Not sleeping well
- Not eating well
- Feeling a bit numb, or fearful, or anxious
- Getting confused or forgetful
- Not coping as well as they used to

Any of these responses may be applicable for family members, as well as someone living with dementia. Regardless, professional support and a health review would be warranted.

My stages of dementia grief – By Robyn
(Wife of husband with dementia)

```
RELIEF - We finally knew what was wrong.
REALITY - The realisation that THIS IS a death sentence.
ANGER - Why is this happening to us?
ANXIETY - How can I do this? I'm not a nurse.
ACCEPTANCE - We cannot change this life we've been dealt.
GRIEF - How can I live without my loved one?
GUILT - Overwhelming feeling of things I should have done
differently and better.
```

Grief, loss, and depression

Grief and depression are different but do have similarities. Both have the potential to lead to feelings of intense sadness, insomnia, poor appetite, and weight loss. For people experiencing grief, these are normal reactions to any loss. While the feelings of loss and sadness can be unbearable, the intensity can change throughout the course of a day and may be triggered in response to certain situations or events. Even throughout the sadness of grief there's an ability to experience moments of happiness.

Depression differs from grief as it's commonly more persistent, with constant feelings of emptiness and despair leaving someone finding it difficult to feel joy or happiness. There can be a focus of internal negative thinking with feelings of being useless and worthless. The feelings of sadness associated with the loss of someone to dementia may never go away completely. If depressive symptoms are ongoing or impact on the way someone lives their life or affects their relationships with others, then it's important to get support or professional help.

No one understands what you're going through like the person going through it too.

-Wendy Hall-

When a heart shatters

A difficult part of supporting someone with dementia is the time when family members are no longer recognised by their loved one. The pillar of strength, the person who supported and was always there for their family, no longer sees the faces they previously remembered. For some family members they soldier on regardless and, for others, this heart-breaking time can result in them finding it too upsetting to continue visiting. This again is a time not acknowledged for the enormity of emotions experienced, the different ways family grieve and the friction and devastation this can cause within families.

There is grief because the person that was loved, and who loved in return, has gone. Yet, the conflict arises with the person still there. Those that surround a family will unlikely realise they're grieving, and so the same support is not forthcoming as it would if someone had died in the physical sense.

How difficult it becomes for children as they gradually lose a parent to dementia, with the other parent living a life in a constant state of crisis, coping from day to day, and they themselves needing an enormous amount of support. Often the roles become reversed, with the children taking on a new role to try to support both parents as best as they know how.

'I just feel like I'm in survival mode and I want my life back. I feel really bad for thinking that way.'

- Wife of husband with dementia –

When 'one size fits all' is never a good fit

Within the health and aged care sector, grief and loss is a conversation we must get better at, to help families feel a normality about what they experience, showing them they're not alone. It's no longer acceptable to leave someone grieving, on their own, for a year, 3 years, 6 years, or for a lifetime. The death of a loved one doesn't release, or relieve, what a grieving family member lives with.

They're not suddenly free to move on with their lives or to pick up where they left off 10 years ago. Family members may not show it on the surface. They may continue to greet others with a warm smile, but many remain trapped in trying to figure out what happened, what went wrong and why their hopes and dreams were so cruelly taken from them.

I still connect with a wife who lost her husband to dementia 10 years ago and I can still hear the sadness in her voice, the raw emotion she continues to live with every day. In many ways it's like he died just last week. To me she epitomises what it is to go it alone, not recognising grief in oneself or having it acknowledged by those that surround her. She was let down in the biggest way possible and rather than be angry, we must learn from these stories and do better for the next person; support them in knowing they don't need to feel guilt for something they're experiencing firsthand. Just because they don't have dementia themselves, they still live with the impact like the person with a diagnosis.

We are positioned now to create a better way forward for families, knowing they don't just stop loving or caring just because someone went into higher supported care, or because memories began to fail, or because they left this world for a hopefully, 'better place'.

The time has come to better prepare families for grieving in a way that doesn't fit the way that many of us have been conditioned to understand. Many of us have gone through life associating grief and loss as the death of a loved one with the definition not necessarily applying to a family member who is still very much alive.

This then becomes a mind shift for families in grieving not only for the person they can no longer be, but for who they represented in the lives of others. It's the sadness for the occasions they can't or will no longer celebrate, for the lost conversations over coffee, for the advice once given, for congratulations and commiserations on life's milestones, for the times they should have been there to lend a hand, for the times they should have been a shoulder to cry on, for the times they should have just been at the other end of the phone.

How do we assist family members in their grieving of the loss of a father, mother, grandfather, grandmother, child, sibling, husband, wife, partner who still stand in front of them? How do we support the guilt felt by families who want to care, are scared to care, don't want to care, have no idea what's even going on? How do we support families who stop coming to visit because they see and feel the judgemental glances from others? How do we help alleviate the guilt of only visiting once a year? The starting point is to stop and ask, 'Why'? And then we create a new way of thinking, a new way to have the conversation and put families back in the driver's seat of their own destiny.

Grief is something that takes time to work through. While everyone finds their own way to grieve, it's important to have the support of friends and family or someone else, and to talk about loss when it's needed.

Melissa's story (continued)...

The diagnosis of dementia impacted Melissa in every aspect of her life. Her career as a teacher was gone, along with colleagues she'd had good support from and spent time with, all who eventually vanished. Her early retirement was a significant loss in her life as her earning potential decreased. Melissa no longer identified as a teacher, and the change to her life now saw her referred to as Tim's carer. Her loss of self-determination was significant.

Family dynamics changed significantly for Melissa, as she transitioned from her role as a wife and mother to mediator and carer. The fracturing of her family was a significant change to her life. The loss of support and feelings of isolation were further exacerbated as her children became estranged and the strong bond and connection she'd had with them previously was now strained. Everyone within the once strong family unit was now going it on their own and grieving all alone.

As Melissa's role as Tim's carer increased, the time constraints became more demanding. Her health regime was difficult to maintain as she devoted more time to caring and navigating through significant life issues. She pushed herself beyond what she could do, she became sleep deprived, her physical health was impacted and her resilience depleted. The couple's life savings were consumed throughout the process. Financial stress impacted Melissa as she struggled to access services and supports suitable for Tim as someone living with a younger onset diagnosis. They were ineligible for many of the services Melissa had reached out to due to Tim's age.

Some people believe that those impacted by dementia can just 'move on' when their loved one dies. The reality is somewhat different. Melissa and Tim's story highlights why this may not always be possible or as easy as it may sound. Many family members are denied the opportunity to work through the complexities of grief and loss as they appear through the lens of dementia, and this is likely from time of diagnosis through to time of bereavement.

Supporting someone experiencing grief and loss

If you are reading this from the perspective of a supporter for a family member who has taken on a care role, the following may provide some ideas for the extended role you play. This highlights the many layers of support needed when someone has a diagnosis of dementia.

It's often difficult to know what to say or do when trying to comfort someone through their grief. It's even more challenging in the case of dementia when those surrounding the person don't easily identify that's what they're possibly going through. If we can increase awareness through ongoing dialogue, then support networks are better placed to offer what families, and someone living with dementia, need most from them.

Sometimes keeping it simple is a good starting point, particularly in an area that many may feel uncomfortable:

- Ask how they're feeling. Take time to listen and understand their perspective and what they're going through.

- Acknowledge what they're likely living with on a day-to-day basis and how hard that must be while avoiding offering solutions or suggestions.

- Be genuine and honest – 'I'm not sure what to say or do, but I want you to know I am here for you'.

- Be ongoing with your offer of support. Every day will be different and bring new challenges – 'What can I do to help? Do you feel like talking?'. Provide options of home cooked meals, doing the shopping, or even going for a walk. Doing something enjoyable together may also help give someone a sense of time out from what they're experiencing.

- Avoid statements that are intended to provide comfort but actually minimise the experience of grief.

- Offer comfort as families will need to feel supported in their loss.

- Feel comfortable with silence, accepting how helpful it can be at times just to offer comfort by a squeeze of the hand, a reassuring hug, or sharing a cup of tea.

- Silence may offer family members time to gather their thoughts and reflect on times gone by.

- Be patient, sit and listen as stories of loss and sadness are shared and expressed.

- Talk about everyday life too. Often families and the person with dementia themselves seek a sense of normality in conversations.

- Encourage them to seek professional support if grief doesn't seem to ease over time.

(adapted from Beyond Blue help sheet - 2021)

Preparing for a better tomorrow ...

What could you do to help others share in what life is like for you ......?

Family perspective ...

'To remember the fear in your loved one's eyes, is the reason the tears swell up in yours.'

-Wife of husband with dementia-

Just remember that ...

You grieve because you loved, you were loved, you belonged, and then in a twist of fate, you suddenly felt unloved, that you no longer belonged, and were made to experience the ultimate loss that is dementia.

-Wendy Hall-

4 • Planning for tomorrow

'Family members of terminally ill patients often have unmet needs for communication of information by healthcare professionals and like staff have a poor understanding of the dementia trajectory.'

- Stirling et. al., 2014 p.338

Imagine ...

Imagine when families and the person with dementia have a plan in place for the future with certainty and empowerment and a feeling of moving forward.

In any other area of life, we prepare for what's to come. We put a plan in place that may need adapting, but it's one that at least gives us an idea of how we'll tackle many of life's challenges.

Nobody said there'd be a mountain

As families start their journey down the dementia road, leading them into the unknown, they soon realise that although they're on the right road they're not actually sure where it's heading.

Many will begin questioning where their ultimate destination will be and how long it will take to get there. It's like being in a small sedan with no supplies because firstly, no one told you to take anything and secondly, you're not sure what it is you should have packed. You head off feeling anxious, not knowing what lies ahead, what might be waiting for you around the next corner.

You drive for a while and things seem to be going smoothly. The sun is shining brightly. Suddenly the road conditions and scenery start to change. What was, at the beginning, a smooth road is suddenly full of potholes. It's not long until the road turns to dirt and now resembles more of a 4-wheel drive track. The road gets steeper as it winds through the mountains. The small and ill-equipped car needs to work harder and harder. The higher you go, the roads become icy, and snow begins to fall. The temperature drops and it begins to get colder.

You weren't given a map and lack the skills and knowledge needed to navigate the ever-changing terrain. The scariest part is there hasn't been any point where you could pull over or turn back. You've committed to the journey and there's no option but to continue forward. You travel for what seems like forever when you finally see a spot to pull over.

You were becoming concerned because without an opportunity to pull over, and refuel, the vehicle would have nothing more to give. It would have just stopped, leaving you stranded and unable to get you to your destination. You pay for fuel and ask for directions, but the person just smiles and tells you you'll be fine, reminding you to rest along the way, if you can. This advice, while well-meaning, doesn't help prepare you for the uncertainty of the road that still lies ahead.

You don't want someone to take over the driving. What you need is someone to point you in the right direction, to help mentally prepare you for what's coming up around the next corner and to share what lies ahead when the road ultimately comes to an end. You want someone who can advise on what to pack and what should be in your toolkit in the possible event of a crisis.

But most importantly what you need, even before starting the journey, is someone who prepared you well ahead of time for the conditions and potential changes you will likely come across. You want someone who has driven down the road before and knows the hazards you will face and ideas about how you might go about navigating these.

Putting a plan in place sooner rather than later ensures no one travels alone, that they're better positioned for timely decision making and not put on the spot, being expected to make time critical decisions in the heat of the moment, and at times when everyone is emotionally charged. This continues to be a heavy weight and an unfair burden for families to have to carry on their own.

Families need to be offered an opportunity to plan and prepare for the more difficult days ahead in a time of calmness and within a peaceful environment. They need to have the chance to talk about what the future could look like, having conversations and putting together ideas that encompass the wishes of the person with dementia themselves, especially if they are still able to contribute.

Families should be empowered to write their own script for their own future. Unless someone like a Dementia Doula is comfortable in having these difficult conversations, families will continue going it alone and suffer in silence. Dementia

Doulas are well positioned to better place families in control of their own destiny, being able to say with conviction, 'This is absolutely what we don't want. These are the things we must have and the things we as a family would be willing to compromise on.'

This includes how care will unfold and what it will look like, where it will take place, through to what the person wants on their toast and how many sugars they have in their coffee. Dementia Doulas don't leave families in a situation where they are just left at the mercy of a disease that has no right to be calling all the shots or dictating how lives will be changed and futures will unfold.

Planning for tomorrow is about no longer telling families what to do, but instead asking them the direction they want to take, presenting them with the information available in a digestible form that they can get their heads around with relative ease – no convoluted jargon, no acronyms and with no assumptions of prior knowledge as to how dementia care and support works. Family members should expect to be asked, 'What can we do for you and how could we go about making it happen?' They should then, with guidance, pick it up from there.

In tribute to ...

In loving memory of Robyn Cutts, always remembered by her children, Sarah, Simon and Vanessa.

Dear Medical Team,

My mum's name was Robyn. She was a registered nurse, a mum, a grandmother, and a wife. She died from Lewy Body dementia. Mum was a fierce lady who wasn't afraid to speak up for herself and felt that she had a good handle on how to manage medical emergencies in our family. Her interest in medicine and caring for others was passed on to both myself, and my sister, with both of us becoming allied health professionals, one a physiotherapist and the other an occupational therapist. Despite our sense of comfort with how to navigate the health and aged care systems, we all failed dismally when it came to providing a good outcome for Mum.

Lewy Body dementia is characterised by psychological symptoms, such as depression, anxiety, paranoia, and hallucinations. Mum started to show signs of finding it difficult to make decisions on simple things and was very anxious. My siblings and I had tried to gently encourage her to seek help, but she refused. The crunch day came when she returned from an overseas holiday and became completely lost when she landed in transit in Sydney. My sister and I received a call from an airline staff member asking if we knew her and where she was meant to be going. They helped us to get her back to Adelaide. She arrived very confused, anxious, and lost. This event became the impetus to convince mum to seek help and we went to her GP.

We were thinking this was going to be our chance to finally start to understand what was going on for mum and work through a plan on how to help her. Unfortunately, the GP was very dismissive and told my sister and I that Mum likely had dementia and we should 'just go home and get her affairs in order'. We asked for a referral to a geriatrician and the memory clinic, but he refused and said, 'You will never get in, the wait list is too long.' I now know that is not true.

Mum didn't seek any further advice and eventually moved to Queensland with my dad. Talking with her on the phone was challenging, with her paranoia increasing. She thought my dad was having an affair with their 100-year-old neighbour! Mum was hallucinating and started to talk about 'the men in the backyard at night who move things around all the time.' When I asked her more about this she shut down and became defensive. I contacted her GP in Queensland who, despite privacy rules, thankfully let me speak to her about my concerns for Mum. The GP convinced Mum to be admitted to the local private hospital under the care of a geriatrician for assessment. Finally, proper tests were undertaken, and she was given a diagnosis of Lewy Body dementia. As an RN, Mum knew what this meant and was worried.

Whilst in hospital, Mum had significant hallucinations that there was a man in her room trying to hurt her. She was very distressed and trying to do everything she could to get out of the room. She was prescribed an antipsychotic medication and the bottom half of her door was locked to stop her from leaving. Nobody thought to take her for a cup of tea, to another space, to let her calm down, or sit with her to reassure her, or a range of other non-pharmacological strategies that may have worked. My sister and I raised our concerns about the use of the anti-psychotic drug being used and its known risks for someone with Lewy Body dementia. We were reassured it was a very low dose and the risk was minimal.

Mum moved into residential aged care and was well cared for and enjoyed it for a week or two but then started to develop an uncontrollable urge to move. She would walk and walk all day and walked herself down to 36 kgs in weight. She was in pain and distress. We would talk via

Facetime, and she would ask me to 'make it stop'. My sister and I asked for help from the GP and the nurses, asking for a specialist review, as we were concerned she had developed akathisia (a side effect of the anti-psychotic medication). We were told that, 'No-one will come to the nursing home.'

Eventually mum started to fall. One awful weekend, I was at my son's football game in Adelaide and was called by the RN at the nursing home in Queensland. She told me mum had fallen and showed me via Facetime a very large, very black bruise on her hip. She was concerned that Mum may have broken her hip. She asked me what I thought she should do. I was shocked, angry, and frustrated. I was in Adelaide, 2000 kms away and she was asking me what to do! I told her my suggestion was that if she thought mum had broken her hip, she required medical attention in hospital and perhaps she could call an ambulance. I then flew to Queensland.

Mum passed away 8 weeks after her initial diagnosis. If she had been diagnosed with cancer, she would have received testing to know what type of cancer she had, an understanding of the prognosis and would have received advice on treatment options. She probably would have been connected to a specialist team who were experts in that specific cancer. Instead, her dementia diagnosis came with no specificity of what type of dementia she had, a lack of care or concern on how to manage it and a lack of knowledge around contemporary treatment options.

Like many cancers, dementia is a life limiting disease that requires a careful palliative approach. My mum received very little support to reduce the significant distress she was in at the end of her life. People living with dementia deserve as much right to a good death as any of your other patients. Provide them with evidence based, person centred and empathetic palliative care.

As a medical profession, please take the time to develop an understanding of the different types of dementia, their presentation, and treatments. Give your patients time and understanding and link them up to the many support services available. Your patients with dementia come from a life of experience, take the time to get to know them. Knowing them will help you to know how to treat them. Following Mum's death, I joined Dementia Support Australia as a Dementia Consultant. If only I knew then what I know now….

From Sarah

Where there's a will there's more certainty

Many people are reluctant or frightened to discuss their end-of-life wishes and this is in part due to the clinical way it's often done or structured. It's a topic that can easily be put off for another day. Formalising important wishes too often gets put on the 'to do' list and for many that's where it ultimately stays. There's also a societal reluctance and stigma attached to talking about death and dying or in looking too far ahead.

The sad reality is, if these conversations don't happen for all of us, regardless of whether someone has dementia or not, when an unanticipated turn of events occurs and there's nothing formalised in place, it means others will need to step up and make life altering decisions on our behalf. These decisions may be in reference to medical treatments we would or wouldn't normally consent to, through to whether we drink tea or coffee.

This scenario has the potential to leave any of us being a passive bystander watching how our lives will play out. I'm sure that's not want any of us want and something that can be easily remedied when addressed early enough.

When advance care plans or directives aren't in place, families are often asked what their wishes are during times of heightened distress and chaos. The reality is, these are important conversations that will happen at some stage regardless of whether they've been previously discussed or not. The unfortunate part is a necessary conversation coming across as insensitive purely due to difficult timing.

When conversations have been previously had, families have a document to default to without feeling pressured to make decisions or think about what's important when they may not feel they have the capacity to do so. When someone's dementia advances, and they lose mental capacity, it will ultimately be up to their next of kin to provide guidance as to the person's wishes about how things should proceed.

As a Dementia Doula, I want to ensure my clients have choices, that they know what their options are, and feel a sense of relief that the decisions they make for themselves or someone they're supporting have been captured, ensuring the wishes reflect the person with dementia as an individual and will bring a sense of dignity to a life still being lived.

Documenting wishes, likes and dislikes isn't just about one area, it covers anything that will influence the well-being of the person and will include environmental considerations as well as what comfort care means and looks like to them as an individual.

The ultimate goal is supporting the person with dementia in experiencing a peaceful life surrounded by those closest to them with four key areas of care being addressed. These include physical comfort, mental and emotional needs, along with spiritual needs.

Gathering up the things that matter ...

For many of us, there's no one else who truly knows what our wishes are or would be down to the finite detail. If we have contributed to what plan A might look like for us in a specific scenario, then we also may need to suggest a plan B or C should things not go the way we thought they might.

If something was to change in our lives tomorrow that meant we couldn't speak or advocate for ourselves then who would know what the plan was? Who would it be that stepped up and got the ball rolling? We don't need to know all the answers to these questions, but we do at least need to have started the conversation with someone we trust. By even talking out loud about this with someone may at least bring some clarity to the situation, so we can consider what is important to us and if we did have the ability to steer the ship, where would we want it to head?

No one within the care sector is a mind reader, although, at times, this would be a useful skill to have. It's up to the person with dementia and their family themselves to write the script for moving forward. Encourage anyone you support to work together, including the person with dementia if appropriate, and go through these questions in a way that will provide an insight into their world, allowing others with more formalised services the opportunity to better connect.

- What do you want others to know about your family member?

- What do you want from others in relation to their care?

- How could others best try and connect and communicate with your family member?

- What is important to them?

- What are the things that help make them feel calm?

- Do you have any advance care plans or advance care directives in place? If yes, where are they located?

- Are they known to others? If so, who?

- What would you want/need from others during stressful times?

Responses don't need to follow any script and may be short or long. It really doesn't matter. They should be reflective of both the person with dementia and the family member themselves. The important part of this process is to just make a start. When this information is captured in a more formalised way, it ultimately becomes a living document, one that can be adjusted, photocopied, changed, or added to at any time. The very knowledge that such a document exists can bring a sense of comfort to those it applies to and an insight to those who can incorporate it into their care practice.

When more support is needed

Transitions through specific stages are an inevitable part of dementia and preparing for them is essential. Without anything in place for how families want to navigate these times, they usually end up going it alone, making it up as they go along and are often at the mercy of available services. These are the times that Dementia Doulas need to ensure families are empowered in the choices they make for their family member with dementia and themselves, that with guidance they are the ones influencing the direction they need to go. They can assist them to navigate this new world they face which is often like nothing they've ever known before.

When families are prepared for what's to come through earlier discussions, the time for more supported care can be navigated in a way that minimises pressured decision making. Without planning, this is a time that leaves families feeling distressed, with minimal options available and decisions needing to be made within days. By having everyone on the same page earlier, there's more opportunity for comprehensive research to be done on services that exist, finding the ones that will meet the needs of the person with dementia, and those that welcome family and their input. Better preparation in this space means the transition into care has a better chance of being done as smoothly as possible.

By better understanding and recognising the stages and symptoms of dementia, families are better placed in anticipating sooner when processes may need to start being put in place. Without this coordinated approach, viable and suitable care options may not be available when they're required.

When a home is not a home

I recall the time my family moved in with a relative while our house was being built. We stayed for an extended period of time and felt immense gratitude for the roof we had over our heads. Everything went smoothly and we always felt comfortable and welcome. However, I also recall feelings of disconnection during this time. It took me a while to realise I was homesick, even though I felt very much at home in my temporary environment. It just wasn't my home.

While I was happy to be there, I likened my experience to going away on holiday, a time where we effectively push the pause button on our normal everyday life. We enjoy our time away, have fun and see life from a different perspective. It's a time to explore new worlds, experience different cultures, have meals regularly prepared and served to us. But there still comes a time when home is at the forefront of our mind, a time where we think the experience has been great but now it's time to go home.

With this comes the anticipation of looking forward to reconnecting with one's space, away from the world, to regroup, resume a 'normal' life and sometimes to go through a period of recovery from the intense time away. Holidays can sometimes come with a hustle and bustle, sightseeing, being constantly on the go, and as enjoyable as that may be, we know it's time to go back to a simpler life with routine and things that we can personally connect with.

Likewise, it can be very confronting and confusing for someone living with advancing dementia moving into supported care, to be told this is your home now, knowing in your heart that isn't really the case. To know that although this is where you now find yourself living, your home is somewhere else. The interesting part to this is that 'home' doesn't have to mean a physical structure, but it does mean a feeling, a place where your heart knows it can rest and be itself.

There have been a couple of times when I've travelled on holidays, where I've come across a place that my heart just connected with: a place where I knew that if I stopped there long enough, I could call it home.

I think when using the term 'home' or creating such an environment for someone with dementia, we need to think about where feeling 'at home' sits for us. In doing so, we're better placed to bring it to life for others to connect with. We ultimately want those that can't physically go home for whatever reason to know we'll influence their space to become the home their heart longs for. Often when someone is reflecting on home and wanting to go home, they may even be referring to a home they'd known as a child, one that at some stage in their long-term memory was a place of comfort, security and where they felt like they belonged.

Take a moment to think about planning for the future ...

- How can we better support someone with dementia as they approach times of transition, particularly into higher supported care? What might these stages look like, how are they identified and how are they best navigated?

- What services are needed compared to the services that appear to be offered? Are they meeting the mark that's needed to fully prepare for all that's to come?

- How prepared should families be in navigating the path they wish to take?

- When preparing someone to transition into higher supported care, what would need to be in place to make this time a natural and seamless experience for all involved?

- What specific social supports and networks do families need surrounding them at this time and how could these be captured and enabled?

As families and the person with dementia enter this new and disorientating environment that is higher care, they are met by a new set of faces of those they must now try to connect with. There's an urgency around getting the person with dementia settled as quickly as possible so business can resume as usual.

This process can change and become more personalised when families know what it is they want and what they're asking for. It's at this point we can also influence the role care staff play by guiding them with the information they need to create an environment conducive to comfort and connection and to be who the person needs them to be.

Monique's story ...

In coming across Wendy's books, I couldn't be more grateful. Not only did I read them and say yes, yes, yes to so many of her ideas on care and life for someone living with dementia, but I also learnt critical information that I had 'no idea' we needed to know.

One such detail was that of the term 'active treatment'. I had yet to raise the subject of an advance care directive with my own mum and dad, but after reading Annette's story in 'The Dementia Doula' and learning what the impact of not understanding the implications of what 'active treatment' could be, I knew we had to get onto it. In broaching the subject with mum, and prior to going through the process of putting her and dad's advance care directives in place, I delicately shared Annette's story.

This made it easier for me to explain the term 'active treatment', making it, I believe, easier for Mum to understand and then making a more informed decision for her and Dad.

The sharing of other people's stories can be so powerful, they can uncomplicate things, make it easier to understand and even be a support in making difficult and sometimes scary decisions.

Preparing for a better tomorrow ...

What could you do to help the person settle more smoothly into a new environment ......?

Family perspective ...

'I'm scared that if he goes into respite for too long that I'll resent him coming back.'

- Wife of husband with dementia –

Just remember that ...

Advanced care planning isn't about checking out next week, or even next month, it's about getting everyone onboard today knowing they're then on the same page when the time comes.

-Wendy Hall-

5 ∘ Connections and reflections

'Another way of maintaining the other's personhood is evidenced by the 'tell me about it' narratives—grandchildren invite their grandparents to recount the past and in the process to reaffirm who they were and still are ... '

- Miron et. al., 2019, p.1034

Imagine ...

Imagine when everyone involved in the care of someone with dementia are better prepared for truly connecting with the person themselves rather than trying to constantly battle the dementia they live with.

Beyond the politeness and the pleasantries lie conversations just waiting to happen, dialogue brewing over many months and years with no place to safely land. Families and support providers turn up every day, going through the motions with no one truly seeing or acknowledging what lay often just below the surface for them, the challenges, conflicts, sadness, and despair.

As we explored in chapter 4, change will only come from better preparing families sooner rather than later or whenever initial contact is made for the future questions they'll likely be faced with and the answers they'll need to have on standby. Without this preparation, families flounder and find themselves lost, trying to find their way around a world that, even many of us working in it, also find difficult to navigate.

Difficult conversations are part of the territory but can only happen effectively when compassionate care principles are in place and enacted. Setting the scene for families for the care expected and support to be received, help them see the role they may or could play moving forward.

As Dementia Doulas, the compassionate care principles we use in our practice assist us in forming relationships with families and someone living with dementia. It's care that's provided based on empathy, respect, and dignity. For staff within the aged care industry who practise compassionate care instinctively, it brings with it an opportunity to form bonds at a much deeper level.

It creates empowerment on both sides and provides those who are influenced by it the chance to flourish and grow into newly defined roles, to be a part of change that can only be possible through the existence of an open dialogue and honesty for where things are heading. For many, there's often a fear within of what they may face and whether they're up to the task.

'I never know how to say goodbye ...'

\-   Granddaughter –

Keeping everyone on board

Staying in touch and connected isn't always easy. Often family members are at different stages of acceptance as they struggle to come to terms with the impact dementia has on a family member and how these changes will affect the family unit. Keeping everyone informed and updated can be a juggling act which may result in family members being lost along the way.

Fractures often form early within family units, not because family members don't care, but more from a sense of grief and loss they themselves are trying to navigate, trying to find their place in the unfolding story, trying to work out what it all means for them. Vanessa shares her story of the challenges she faced early in her dad's diagnosis of dementia. It's a story that's inspiring in its simplicity, as she struggles to keep her family together in the only way she could think of.

Vanessa's story ...

When Dad was given his diagnosis of Alzheimer's it was confirmation of what we, as a family, had been suspecting for more than 12 months. At the time, being the eldest of three sisters, the indirect carer for Mum who has multiple mental health challenges and a support for Dad as Mum's carer, I quite quickly became the 'carer, supporter and advocate' for both Mum and Dad.

I naively thought that the needs of Mum and Dad would be able to be shared between my sisters and me, but that unfortunately was not to be, and I know that it was very much due to our family relationships being quite complex and disconnected due to a lifetime of impact from our mum's mental health challenges. One of the hardest things was managing the communication of what was happening and what was needed by everyone. I would diligently call each sister to either give them an update or to re-clarify conversations they had had with Mum, which would cause more angst and worry than was warranted. Then there were the phone calls to ask for help/assistance that would often be met with push back and me taking back the request for help to minimise conflict. As changes in Dad increased so did the number of calls.

It was one afternoon when I was messaging to a friend who was overseas on WhatsApp that I thought, why don't I just set up a WhatsApp group for my sisters and me. My thinking was that this would allow me to easily share any information with them quickly. Everyone would receive the information at the same time (saving me having to think of, 'Who did I call first last time?'), and if a group call was needed, I could easily make a 3-way call.

So, giving myself a pat on the back I set up a group and messaged both of my sisters to share my idea and how it would work. One sister thought it was a good idea and the other couldn't understand why we needed such a group, leaving me thinking, well, maybe this idea won't work after all? But in not being able to think of another way that I could easily and simply communicate quickly, I decided to stick with the 'Sister's Group'. At first messages were acknowledged but as time progressed more information was asked for, more interest was taken and I think there was more understanding of what was happening and what was needed.

On reflection one day, I wondered if by sharing information this way, it actually gave time and space for my sisters to read and take in the information at a time that fitted them and their own busy lives? For whatever reason it was working and made sharing of information easier.

The 'Sister's Group' started to take on a life of its own. Not only was it about Dad and Mum, but it also evolved, and we started to share other things happening in each of our own lives. Sometimes there may not be any messaging for a number of weeks, but when there is news to be shared or a critical event happens, such as when Dad was admitted to hospital, I was quickly able to communicate what was happening and then confirm the best time for a joint call between us all easily.

Connecting without the normal cues

With other conditions such as a stroke or a broken limb, the visible effects of a plaster cast or paralysis can clearly be seen. Without a second thought, we adapt our expectations of what the person can now achieve with the limitations they're experiencing. We're more accommodating in our approach. Living with dementia creates similar challenges for someone, but the effects can't visibly be seen. Dementia is a physical disease of the brain, and it's only when a person's brain is scanned, that the impact can be realised.

Because we can't see the damage that's occurring to the brain itself, connection with someone with dementia becomes more challenging. Without the visual cues of the damage dementia does, we often take the person at face value and either raise the bar of expectation or keep it firmly raised to the level it had always been. When supporting someone with dementia, I have always attempted to imagine what a dementia plaster cast might look like. It's something tangible I can use to frame my own thoughts that dementia isn't the person, it's something that keeps the person from us.

I envision an actual barrier, almost like a large shield floating in front of the person, making it more difficult for the person to connect with us and for us to connect with them. I picture this barrier as something we've all tried to break through at some stage, with no success. We put pressure on the person to try just that bit harder, reminding them of things we think they should know. We try and assist them to make sense of the world around them, but this too is blocked by dementia every time.

We need to acknowledge and make peace with the fact we can't get through dementia. We can't infiltrate the impenetrable barrier it creates. Over time it becomes too powerful a force. Dementia hides the person that is known and loved by those around them, so rather than trying frustratingly to battle it, we need to sneak around the edges and find another way in, a different and more creative way to connect, one that dementia has no way of stopping.

Becoming more creative with how we connect with the person may take a bit more effort on our part but, it will always be worth it. Living with dementia must leave the person feeling deflated, tired of fighting from the inside, constantly trying to get their messages across to us, but not being understood in the way they now express themselves. But learning the person's new language in some form will bring a whole new meaning to the connections that are made.

You'll never know unless you ask

When connecting with family members, our questions must be carefully considered and come with an option for not having to respond. I was grateful for the following responses from Cath who supports her husband Michael with dementia. Her honest and open insights to the questions asked provide us all with a snapshot into their world. By Cath being candid, those that surround them in everyday life are then better equipped to meet them both where they're at:

What has Michael taught you about getting through each day?

Patience, patience, patience. Going with the flow, going slower, not feeling bad about asking for help. How to keep an eye on my tone when I get frustrated with him. To be less fussed about how I would usually have done things, for example, asking Michael to hang out the clothes on the line – and not caring how they are hung… no pegs and all skewwhiff.

What has Michael taught you from your shared experience?

Oh, so much – how much I love him most of all….

What support might have made your path just that bit smoother?

I think understanding in more detail how sexually things change… both partners still have wants or needs and not quite sure how to traverse this without feelings of inadequacy occurring.

Who supported you when you needed it most and what did that look like?

Oh, my goodness – I have a whole village all over the world helping us via Messenger. Friends in the UK and interstate are always there for a chat or a message when it's difficult. There are 2 dedicated group chats to check how things are going, where I can go to rant and who can come to me at a moment's notice if needed.

Our church community - especially one couple who invite us to join them with things they know Michael will manage and feel comfortable with, including meals out and at home, weekends away, cups of tea, visits… The rest of the church community especially six others are also available for a walk, an outing, a drink, either just with Michael or with us both.

Our family - Michael's son travels for an hour every Wednesday to come and have tea with us and spend time with his dad. Michael is always happy and proud and somehow comforted after he's visited for those 2 hours. Michael's sister takes him out weekly for a couple of hours for a cuppa. It's always on the same day so he always knows it's Monica's day on a Thursday.

My sister is there for me, whether it be for a walk, getting our nails done together, taking Michael out when another arrangement falls through and, who listens at any time to my concerns, upsets, frustrations, sadness, happiness. His cousins are a little band of pure gold. They are 3 couples who live across Adelaide and South Australia. We have weekends away with them. They take him out, just the boys, and make sure he's included. They care for him with toileting, eating etc and making light of it all.

My friends care for me, taking me out, sometimes not asking too many questions, sometimes asking just the right question, and coping with me being late or flustered to our planned breakfast. Other friends, who seem to have come out of the woodwork, take Michael out weekly or are a stopgap measure for lunch and a walk. They pick him up, manage his belongings, help with ordering food, paying for the food, help with managing utensils and toileting.

And then there's a mixed bag of people who are on my list of 'can call for help'. I just have to refer to it and see what I need and who could help. I feel very blessed.

A note to myself:

To remind myself of parts of our recent trip to the UK. A friend had offered to do a trip with us. I wouldn't have considered going at all, but we did. After all the preparation, we arrived safely at the airport and Monica (Michael's sister) came to see us off shouting us all a Buck's Fizz cocktail. How special! She said she'd seen Michael off on his first overseas trip many years ago and thought this might be his last - poignant yet fabulous that our mate Helen helped enable this. xx

So, we've set off on the first leg of our trip, very excited, but found myself crying a little from my wonderful business class pod (which was our only option for Michael to travel feeling emotionally comfortable). As I look across, I can see Michael struggling with his meal. His steak is all cut up, but he can't manage the knife with serrations pointed down. It's so sad the disease takes so many things away from a person.

Anyway, he's so happy and Helen set him up with watching Downton Abbey… so all happy and calm. I'm a bit anxious that nothing too serious goes wrong, so I suggested 4 alcoholic drinks was enough for Michael, 1 in the airport, 1 before take-off, and 2 glasses of red with his meal.

Michael seemed happy enough with the arrangement but was cross about it later… hum...

By Cath …

A considered approach

Before attempting to connect with anyone, we must always consider our approach. Approach often sets up for the intended connection we're hoping to make. If there's a strong tone in a person's voice, we think we're in trouble. If the person is extra nice to us, we know they want something from us.

Think about arriving home and as you approach your front door, it swings open. You're greeted by the warmest of welcomes and the person you reside with offers to take your coat. They validate that you've likely had a full-on day and reassure you they have a cup of coffee and a cheese platter waiting for you to relax and unwind.

This scenario is full of wonderful intentions and gestures. It's intended to make us feel like someone cares about us, but what this act inadvertently does is push our suspicion radar button. You see, we're not used to others being 'extra' nice to us for no good reason. We're instantly suspicious of their motives. We may even think along the lines of, what have they done, what do they want, or how much is this going to cost me? Approach becomes everything.

If we approach someone in a rushed manner or with our thoughts elsewhere, the person will feel it. They'll sense we're not really in the moment with them and may be reluctant to share their thoughts or how they're feeling. Someone living with dementia is no different. If they sense a disinterest in someone's body language or tone of voice, then any sort of connection will be near impossible. If a voice in any way sounds condescending, that too will shut down any hope of meeting the person where they're at.

Whenever I've wanted to connect with someone in any setting, I've found myself trying to picture myself in their shoes, to think about the situation they find themselves in and try to connect with that experience. For example, during my paramedic days, I would create a picture in my mind and think about how frightening it would be to be woken up in the middle of the night, in my own bed, in my own bedroom within my own home. Things would be happening so fast and as I would try to open my eyes, I'd be blinded by the light someone had switched on. All I would be able to see would be the silhouette of 2 or 3 people standing next to me or at the end of my bed.

With or without my glasses on I would find it difficult to focus, to work out what they're saying and why they're in my bedroom. Who might they be? They would all likely be talking at the same time and all I would be able to pick up on is an authoritative voice instructing me to do something.

I know I don't wake easily and would find this situation difficult to navigate. I would be frightened and wondering how they got into my room in the first place. My autopilot response would likely be to defend myself, to tell them to get out, to resist them trying to get me out of bed.

I pictured this scene and relived this scene many times in my mind throughout my career. It was a scenario that would ground me on a call in the middle of the night, to a house where someone may not be expecting us or even if they were. I would think back to how overwhelming that would feel if it was happening to me. It changed my thinking, made me consider my approach, and it changed how I connected with the person. The rules remain the same regardless of whether someone has dementia or not and I still find it useful today.

Liz's story …

While inviting family members to contribute to this edition, I encouraged those who were not sure what to write to perhaps consider writing a letter to hopefully make sharing their experiences in written form just that bit easier. On returning her letter, Liz shared that before sending her letter back, she first sent the letter to her adult children to read and ensure they felt comfortable with what she was sharing and putting out there.

Liz was surprised that they were not only okay with what she had written but also commented that they'd had no idea that was how she'd felt. It had been many years since Liz had lost her husband and her children their beloved father, and while time had passed, the importance of writing that letter and sharing it with them had not been lost. Carrying the weight of dementia doesn't just go away just because the person has died.

The power of the written word

A letter is often an opportunity to express a range of feelings and emotions, to share disappointments and triumphs, to celebrate special occasions and reminisce about times gone by. They have historically been an important part of our societal fabric and one that makes time and distance melt away, where two people can be joined not in person but through the sharing of words.

Words don't always come easily, especially when we're not feeling comfortable with a topic or within a certain context, or when there's a lack of confidence with a particular subject. But when writing a letter, sometimes the words flow more easily, giving us a chance to tap into feelings rather than thinking and wondering whether they're the right words to use.

While compiling material for this book, I invited family members to write a letter to the person they support or supported, one that may never be read or never be sent. But it could be one of the most important letters they have ever written.

A letter will always find its intended audience, even if that turns out to be the author themselves. A letter provides an opportunity to write from the heart without the pressure of a story line or word count. It can capture feelings and meanings that may never have been previously recognised or acknowledged.

As the words often flow freely, letters provide an opportunity to reflect, to slow things down, to think from the heart in a way that words won't always convey. As a daughter shared after writing a letter about the experience of supporting her mother with dementia, 'I didn't realise I'd write so much. There was lots I didn't realise I needed to say. I think it was the letter I needed to write to let go of a lot of stuff I didn't realise was just sitting there'.

Quite often, the path we seek and the answers we are searching for are hidden behind the complexities of the moment, the stiffness of a situation, the blinding nature of language used towards and at us that may not be inclusive.

Families are often left feeling alienated from the new world they are attempting to discover and navigate. Through the act of letter writing, there are no rules or expectations, just a freedom to be who someone needs to be in that given moment.

'I don't want others to think I just gave up on him.'

- Wife of husband with dementia –

Ann-Marie's story ...

Ann-Marie sent through this beautiful moment she shared in after better understanding her mum's lived experience with dementia.

Ann-Marie lives interstate from her parents and rang her mum (who has dementia) to wish her happy birthday. Her father put her mum on the line, and she said, 'Hi Mum, it's Ann-Marie here. I'm just ringing to say happy birthday'. Her mother replied with, 'My mum, did you say my mum, where's my mum, my mum's dead?'. Ann-Marie then replied with a slow and pronounced voice, 'No, you are my mum and it's your birthday'. Her mum replied, 'Where did you say my mum was?'.

Ann-Marie took a moment along with a deep breath and reflected on the first book of this series – *'Dementia can't take everything!'*. She remembered how overwhelming conversation for someone with dementia can become, especially when we use too many words and attempt to prompt a memory the person clearly doesn't connect with.

And with her considered reply simply said, 'I love you Mum', to which her mum replied 'Oh, that's lovely dear'. A simple statement with a big impact. By keeping her messaging simple, a connection was powerfully made.

Preparing for a better tomorrow ...

What could you do today to make tomorrow a little easier ......?

Family perspective ...

'Makes me sad knowing what mum needs but not knowing how to make it happen...'

– Daughter –

Just remember that ...

Perception of dementia starts with the words we use, the actions we take, the dignity and respect we show, and the environment we create within which others can grow.

-Wendy Hall-

6 • Creative caring

'Memory boxes help stimulate the long-term memory of a person living with dementia.'

- Heath et. al., 2019 p.1

Imagine …

Imagine when families are better equipped with the tools they need for the role they will ultimately play.

Families often want to contribute and do more for the person with dementia but are just not sure what to do or how to go about it. Many feel alienated from decision making and how they should or could integrate themselves within a care environment. By assisting families to build their own visiting toolkits, like we do for our Dementia Doulas in their practice, we place them in a better position for meaningful connections.

By assisting families to be more creative with their connections, the sky becomes the limit for what they can bring together.

They're better positioned for problem solving, finding their own solutions and more enjoyable ways to care. By building the confidence of family members, we reassure them that they still know the person with dementia better than anyone and hold the key to questions being asked by others.

Often what families need is a starting point to capture what brings comfort to the person with dementia, what's important to them and what's most likely to be worrying them and keeping them awake at night.

Families are and always have been the missing link in taking dementia care to the next level. They're the piece of the puzzle we've long been searching for when it comes to knowing who the person with dementia is at the core.

They are an entity with an understated worth for what they ultimately bring to the table. Families can overlook the value of the information they hold, with many feeling their insights spanning a person's lifetime, is not important or relevant in the current context.

There is information that families often perceive as insignificant that can provide staff with a missing link for understanding why someone with dementia is behaving or responding in a specific way. When that information is able to be shared, the opportunities for how it can be incorporated into conversation and care become endless.

The answers to the questions care staff are often looking for may not always be in a current day context. Someone unsettled at night may think they're up waiting for late teenagers to arrive home from a night out or wondering if the doors are locked and the bins out for the morning. For someone with dementia, the priorities from yester year may continue to be priorities today.

Cath shares ...

We have a white board on the kitchen cupboard which I update every evening when Michael's gone to bed. It includes the date and day of the week:

Wednesday 6th February
9am - 1pm choir with Darren
Cath home, then walk with sister
6pm - Will over for dinner

I also have bought a 'dementia clock' which is located in the TV room. It has large lit numbers and includes – morning/afternoon and day of the week. Michael refers to the clock and the white board often.

I try to keep to routines and have things in the same places. I also try to use the same patterns of speech. In the morning I lay his clothes out while he is in the shower. Sometimes he heads back to the bedroom to try and get dressed. At other times he comes through naked to the kitchen not sure what to do.

I send him back and he heads back down the passage to the bedroom. Sometimes he can get his underwear on, other times not and sometimes back to front. We move on, always in the same order, he sits down while I do his socks and shoes. While I'm putting his belt through the trouser loops we sing – 'Turn around' by Cyndi Lauper as he has to turn around.

Getting ready for mealtimes – it's Michael's job to set the table. I usually direct him to the drawer several times and he'll go back and forth several times with 2 forks or 2 knives. I just redirect as I'm preparing the vegetables. Sometimes I hand them to him and he can place them on the placemat. We check it together, then add or delete anything. I always have his pills in a small white dish that he can easily see next to his water glass on the table. We always sit at the table together to eat. This helps with all sorts of things, normality, not too much mess on the floor, a bit of chat, orientation to the mealtime.

Some things are labelled such as the bathroom drawers, and his chest of drawers but I don't really know if that helps at all.

And praise – not empty praise, but real praise such as, 'You were really funny today and made Louise laugh. She does enjoy your company….' I always end the day with, 'Good night. Thank you for a lovely day', as I tuck him in. Then I go back to the TV room to have a couple of hours to myself.

I try to only have one main activity planned for Michael each day. Or if he has two things on, I allow for a rest/sleep/nap for an hour or two in between. I try to get Michael outside with me if I'm hanging out washing or gardening. He can be involved and hold things or pass things to me. There's a stool near the veggie patch where he can come and sit and chat while I work.

If I'm frustrated or upset, I try and use a pleasant tone and I tell him I'm just a bit overwhelmed and going to have 5 minutes to myself and take myself outside. Sometimes I don't tell him and just head outside anyway. He'll always come and find me after 10 minutes or so anyway – and by then I'm good.

Take a moment …

I asked Andrew, who lives with dementia, if he'd be willing to share some stories of his life so we could help others to better understand who he was and where he was coming from. Andrew looked at me with a concerned look on his face said, 'But the only problem is I can't read anymore!'

I gave him a reassuring smile and said, 'That's okay, I don't want you to read or write your story, I just want you to tell your story'. His sighed as he replied, 'Oh, good, that's okay then'.

We can't necessarily change the impact dementia has on a person, but there's nothing stopping us from influencing the small, everyday things that enhance wellbeing and contribute to a better quality of life.

Handing back memories

We often expect people with dementia to remember in the everyday sense like we all do. When they're unable to retrieve a memory, we think the memory is likely now gone along with the ability to recall moments from the past. What is often overlooked is the ability we have to assist people with dementia in remembering times gone by. If we pivot in our approach and stop trying to bring the person to us and meet them where they're at, we in effect hand them back their stories.

I think back to David who was living with dementia and attended many activity groups I was part of. David often appeared most comfortable being on the sidelines. He enjoyed watching others participate. Along with my colleagues, we would capture these precious moments as photos thinking they would one day be valuable for family members to share in. As Christmas approached one year, we made up a slideshow of the photos we'd collected throughout the year. We ran it on loop for families and the person with dementia they supported, to enjoy a snapshot of the year we'd shared together.

What we hadn't anticipated was David's reaction and response to the slideshow. While family members connected, David walked over to the wall with the pictures projected onto it and the look on his face was priceless. It was as if he'd been instantly transported back in time. He smiled from ear to ear and there was a sense of calmness and tranquility.

David became immersed in the year that had been. He recognised himself in photos and while it was unlikely he remembered the actual events firsthand, he appeared to be reliving the moments as they scrolled by. These were not old memories for him, but by using the slideshow as a reminiscence tool, David was transported back in time, his memories handed back to him in a way he could connect with and enjoy a second time around.

Putting together a reflection box

A reflection box may assist families in their recall of events and people from the past. They provide the person with dementia, families and staff the opportunity to look back at memories and keepsakes often thought to be lost in time. They can stimulate and prompt conversations that may never have been previously shared. The simple touch of a seashell or rock, once collected on a holiday, has the capacity to transport everyone back in time, to special moments shared together or with others.

Reflection boxes can be used to promote engagement opportunities for people living with dementia and prompt conversations that create mental and emotional stimulation. For a person living with dementia, the items or objects contained in a reflection box can stir thoughts of happy moments in life and give them something to talk about. Research supports the idea that talking with people living with dementia about their lives can create positive emotional experiences, reduce stress, and provide a better quality of life.

Reflection boxes can help produce these beneficial responses by connecting the person to what makes them feel comfortable and happy. A reflection box should contain a variety of items that hold a special significance for the person with dementia and can be used to engage or comfort them when needed.

Importance of a reflection box

A reflection box gives someone with dementia the possibility of opening up about and sharing in memories from their past. It provides an opportunity for family members and other support providers to gain insights into who the person is and where they've come from. The reflection box should be developed in such a way as to stimulate all the senses including touch, hearing, sight, smell and taste. Research suggests the interactions with a reflection box can assist with improving someone's mood, their self-esteem, and overall wellbeing.

The reflection box can open up and inspire conversations with family members, caregivers, children, or grandchildren. A reflection box provides the opportunity for a meaningful activity for families. They become more creative in their ideas for box design and in the sourcing contents to put in them.

Many years ago, I attended a craft fair with a friend. We stopped at a display containing an assortment of scented hand creams. Each were scents I was familiar with and included lavender, rose, citrus and then I found myself stop at violet. This was a scent I couldn't recall; it was one I was intrigued with as I didn't think it was one I knew. I picked it up to smell and was instantly transported back in time.

In that moment, I was transported back 30 years to the interstate home of my nana just before she died. The memories of visits and how special she'd been to me came flooding back in a flash. I felt wrapped in a sense of comfort I couldn't comprehend. I bought the violet hand cream purely for the memories it elicited in me. I used it on my hands before going to bed each night and could smell it as I fell asleep. The scent would stay on my pillow like a reassuring touch.

Using the senses opens up further opportunities for connecting and can in turn create a safe and comfortable buffer around the person with dementia so they no longer feel alone. Agitation, restlessness, and emotional distress are not uncommon in the later stages of dementia, and the sharing of happy memories through the objects contained within a reflection box may elicit a positive response with calming results.

Ideally someone with dementia should have a box personalised for them based on their life story and containing objects of meaning. If this isn't possible or the person has no one to bring such a box together for them, then a generalised version is an ideal starting point.

The earlier a reflection box is created, the more chance there is of the person with dementia contributing to the content selection and sharing stories that can be captured and documented for future use.

'Saying goodbye is always upsetting for her.'

- Daughter of mother with dementia –

Reasons to create a reflection box

Reflection boxes can link a person with dementia to the things that have most meaning for them and can make them feel good about themselves. They can be a gateway to a person's identity in such a way that they can use the contents to express who they are and be seen more clearly by others without explanation. The opportunity to use such a tool as a form of communication can result in an increase in confidence, self-esteem, and sense of belonging. Using specific themes and objects enables the person with dementia to show others the things that bring them comfort and happiness.

Families have often commented that the more items they searched for, the more life memories came back for them also. The creation of a reflection box provided an often well needed distraction that doubles as a sense of purpose.

Creating a reflection box

The first step in creating a reflection box is locating a suitable container which can take many forms. Options may include a basket, plastic container, ornate bag, shoebox, or gift box. It can be decorative or simple but should be strong, robust and easily stored. A fun activity may be involving young children or grandchildren in the decorating of the box with the person with dementia.

A shoebox is ideal. While being easy to access and lift, it is also able to store several items of reasonable shapes and sizes and fit on someone's lap or side table. If the reflection box has compartments and is designed for access by the person with dementia, consideration should be made for the person's fingers and dexterity. The box will be created for regular and possibly shared use, so ensure it can handle some wear and tear and will open easily.

What to include

The reflection box can contain anything of meaning for someone with dementia and include their previous interests and favourite things. Items stored within a reflection box can be personal, and may seem ordinary, like a blank postcard. They may represent moments in history that have meaning to the person such as royal memorabilia or old stamps.

Keep in mind that the brain doesn't just store visual memories so you might include items with different textures, scents, or sounds. Each item chosen should relate to a memory that can be revisited over and over again. When including things like diaries, letters, and newspaper articles, consider that some items may bring back memories that are distressing or sad.

Sensitivity and reassurance will be needed when the reflection box is being used. Providing an opportunity for the expression of emotions is not necessarily a bad thing, but it is how we respond and react that is significant. The person should not be left alone, and a future consideration may be to remove the items and feedback the findings to other support providers.

Ideas for inclusion in a reflection box

- Holiday souvenirs
- Trophies or medals
- Seashells or small jar of sand
- Letters from a loved one
- Favourite family recipe
- Sheet music or old record of favourite song
- Musical instrument

- Favourite CD
- Keychains
- Postcards
- Toy animal
- Newspaper clippings
- Jewellery
- Old coins
- Hairbrush/comb
- Favorite books or stories
- Family heirlooms
- Christmas ornaments, stockings, or religious items
- Thimble, sewing pattern, cotton spools
- Labelled copies of family photos
- Sporting equipment or memorabilia
- Swatches of different fabric types, textures and colours
- Dried flowers, petals, pinecones, leaves
- Favourite perfume or hand lotion
- Potpourri sachet
- Favourite bar of soap
- Artwork from children or grandchildren
- Gardening gloves

In addition: When copying documents/photos include dates if available and consider laminating items for protection and to highlight specific themes.

Considerations for choosing items

Safety:

Safety is of utmost importance when considering objects for inclusion and if in doubt, leave them out. Collections of smaller items such as seashells are better placed in small, see through or organza type bags. If rings are to be included, they could be tied onto a long piece of ribbon so they can still be held and seen but the risk of choking or getting lost is reduced.

When using valuable items, the reflection box should be brought in only for the time of the visit and taken home again for security reasons. A second box could be made up of less valuable items and left with the person for use by staff or other visitors.

It may prove easier when trying to get back an item from the person with dementia when leaving if it can be substituted with something of greater connection and interest to the person that can be safely left with them.

Avoid any items that are potentially dangerous, precious, heavy, or sharp and if an item is rare or irreplaceable then it should be left out altogether. Items included should be easy to handle and not too heavy.

A family member may consider taping their own fingers together and seeing how easy it is to hold and look at an item before its inclusion. Arthritic fingers that lack dexterity may find certain items cumbersome and painful to hold.

Significance:

When considering items think back to those that are more likely to elicit happy and positive memories. Keep in mind that not all tears are sad ones.

Texture:

The texture of items can also help stir memories, like a piece of satin from a favourite dress, a furry stuffed animal, or a shoe cleaning brush may all trigger sensory memories when held.

Fragrance:

Including items that can be touched and smelt. With altered sensory perception, a person with dementia might not have the same ability to smell like they did but it may be worth a try. For example, a lavender sachet may remind someone of one placed in drawers from many years ago.

Identification:

Someone with dementia may not recognise certain items or understand their significance. Using labels may provide a useful prompt and assist others in initiating conversations about specific items. For example, Grandpa's gardening gloves, Mum's wooden spoon, Betty's necklace. Attach the label directly to the items or use handwritten tags. A list may also be included in the box of all items, along with a short sentence or story about each one.

Using a reflection box

The possibilities for what to include in a reflection box are endless. This is an opportunity for families to come together and to be creative as they collect a variety of memory-stimulating items that are designed specifically for their loved one.

When items have been selected, the person with dementia should be included in the process, encouraging them to handle each item while noting their responses and reactions, and discovering those which resonate for them. Talking about the significance of an item may prompt the person with dementia with their connection and association with it.

Multiple reflection boxes can be created for different themes or occasions and hold different memories for the person. They may include memories of a particular sports team, hobby, religious celebrations, or holiday destination and don't have to all fit into a single box. Multiple boxes mean one can be safely left with the person (for use by staff or other family members), ensuring it doesn't contain items of monetary or sentimental value. It may contain copies of documents, cards and letters and items from a secondhand store if there are concerns about things getting lost or going missing.

A second or subsequent box may contain personal and valued items that are taken into a visit and home again after. Should a person with dementia be holding a treasured item and not wanting to part with it, include something that sparks interest and connection to swap that can be safely left with the person. It's important to not create undue distress for the person when an item is suddenly taken away.

Ethel's story ...

My husband's grandma, Ethel, was in higher care many years ago. For her 90th birthday a small afternoon tea had been organised in the care home café. A cake was provided and next to it stood a red cylindrical candle that would be lit for the obligatory chorus of, 'Happy Birthday'. While Ethel was confused with the transpiring events and wondered who all the people surrounding her were, there was a joy on her face as she thought she was attending a wedding.

A family member presented her with a single stem of 7 orchids. We watched as Ethel held it and viewed it closely. We saw her gently touch the individual flowers and it then appeared as though she was considering ripping them off the stem. A family member was about to stop her when Ethel began speaking in a quiet voice.

Standing closer to her, we could hear her quietly speak. She pointed to what she had considered to be the front of the stem, then she turned the stem around and pointed to the flowers she indicated were, 'Facing backwards and needed to come off'. Without this dialogue and an understanding of her intent, it appeared, at face value, that Ethel was going to destroy the orchid stem and was about to have it taken off her.

We all stood and shared in this special story, as family reminisced about Ethel's days as a flower grower and florist. What she was doing was preparing the stem for a flower bouquet or arrangement. But it didn't stop there, Ethel then began poking the top of the unlit candle with the stem and it didn't take long to then realise she thought the candle was a vase.

By taking a step back, watching how things unfolded and placing Ethel's life story into the unfolding scene, we were able to see not only what was happening, but for just a moment in time we were able to see the world through her eyes.

Preparing for a better tomorrow ...

What could you do that's creative ......?

Family perspective ...

'If we had the knowledge, the endless patience and the correct skills to look after a loved one with dementia, we would also have the cure.'

-Wife of husband with dementia-

Just remember that ...

When I see the creation of a special moment come to life, I will capture it, bottle it up and share it so others may be inspired to do and feel the same.

-Wendy Hall-

7 • Navigating the path as a united front

'Fresh thinking and more resources may be needed to challenge persisting common misapprehension of the condition and the formation of entrenched stigma.'

- Rosato et. al., 2019 p.1

Imagine ...

Imagine when all those surrounding the person with dementia and their families come together in a way that will change life as they know it.

Creating a culture of compassionate care is about opportunities to practice dementia care with respect and dignity. It's not just about better connections with someone with dementia, it's also about uniting everyone involved in the care of the person, while including their families. When creating a united front, a more inclusive care approach can be initiated which offers families a more pivotal and meaningful role in the care provision.

When put into position early enough, a supportive community provides a big soft comfy pillow where family members can safely fall, or where they can rest their heads to escape from the world for a while and absorb the tears that often flow freely. When providing this space and support for families, grief, loss and outpouring of emotions can then run to their own timelines and no longer be squeezed into the timelines of others.

Becoming a supportive community is about honest and open dialogue, with everyone clearly understanding the role they play. It's understanding and listening to the person with dementia and their families, knowing what is important to them at any given time. It's a connection with others that increases the chances of issues being picked up earlier, of approaches being incorporated into care sooner to ensure the ongoing comfort of the person with dementia.

By listening to the frustrations and system shortfalls faced by families in the earlier stages of dementia, an opportunity is created for putting a framework in place that better meets needs in real time. It assists in identifying where wider system shortfalls exist, changes that need to occur and ways these might be fixed. When sharing in the experience of families in identifying, diagnosing, and navigating dementia as a condition, we are not only better positioned to appreciate the actual role families play, but also to understand the role they want to play and the contributions they are willing to make.

From a wife of husband with dementia ...

Dear Medical Staff,

Please give all people diagnosed with dementia dignity and respect. Please communicate with and include the person living with dementia. Do not ignore them. Enable the person to maintain the maximum possible level of independence, choice and control.

Also, please listen to their carer, family, or support person. Be supportive, compassionate, and understanding. Once there is a diagnosis of dementia, you are not just treating one person, but two. The carer needs to be looked after also.

Please understand that from diagnosis, even though this is a terminal disease, the person can still have a very special, wonderful life with many experiences for maybe many years. They do not have to have everything taken away from them now. Assist them to maintain confidence and a positive self-esteem.

Understand medications, and do not over medicate. Many times, "behaviours" can be from frustration at not being able to communicate, being made to do things the person does not want to do, from pain, loneliness, isolation, boredom - just to name a few.

As this is a terminal disease, please support the family with Palliative Care all along their experience.

Thank you,
Jenny - my husband's carer

Research is telling us that ...

It's important that we incorporate more relationship-centred practices into care home settings to ensure that service delivery promotes dignity and compassion. Relationship-centred practices included everyone from families, care staff, clinicians, and the person with dementia themselves. They assist with fostering the building of connection and trust and leave someone with dementia and their family members feeling valued and appreciated.

This compassionate care framework ensures staff can reflect on their everyday practices and identify not only what they're doing but how it impacts others. Opportunities are also created for ensuring the voices of families are heard and their input valued and considered. Ultimately, more positive dementia care experiences result within both community and higher care settings.

'Compassion towards people with dementia is often suboptimal, which can impact negatively on clinical outcomes and care.'

-General Practitioner (GP)-

Keeping families in the loop

It's important moving forward that everyone involved in dementia care has proper, consultative input into what the future of dementia care should look like. This includes staff, families, communities, and the person themselves, all contributing to further models of care that would potentially make a tangible difference to quality of life of the person living with dementia and their families.

Care should also include the development of roles that are missing within the sector, independent of care workers and clinicians all of whom already have enough in their job descriptions to keep them busy in the work they already do.

We've developed the Dementia Doula role to better support families in being more empowered in the role they play, but we know there's many more that need to follow.

By families answering the following type of questions, there's an opportunity to start framing what further roles within the sector could look like. These roles cover priority areas that currently fall by the way due to a lack of time and resources.

Conversations to be captured should be from both the person with dementia and family member perspectives and include:

- Writing a job description for the role that could best support you today, what would that look like?

- In planning for the future, what services would you want in place?

- What support would you want from those services and what would this look like?

- If those services were in place, what would your everyday life look like?

- How could others make you feel supported?

Another useful way to involve families is encouraging them to keep a notebook and write down all the questions they have regardless of whether they're big or small. The notebook becomes their extended memory and is at the ready when opportunities for addressing queries arise. A notebook may also be useful for framing any concerns or needs families may have and they should be encouraged to include insights into what they think is working and what could do with some improvement.

This isn't about catching anyone out in their practice but to enable families to share what they feel and contribute in a way they're prepared for. When family members are asked what they need or want, many will be unable to reply because the shortfalls they face are often absorbed into everyday life.

If families are included and supported in a way that enables them to play a more active role in care provision, they are better connected and involved in everyday decision making and assisted with alleviating or reducing the guilt often experienced.

When families feel a disconnection from the care of their family member with dementia, they may feel ostracised, disempowered, as if their feedback isn't valued or has a place. They can feel like their family member is being treated as a number. The success stories often come from family members who feel valued, comfortable and included, and have an established rapport with staff within a specific environment.

Michael's story ...

Michael lives with dementia. He's a natural born storyteller and when he takes a big deep breath and slowly exhales says, "Wellllll", I know I need to sit back and buckle up because a big story will shortly follow.

I always smile in anticipation of his stories. I don't think it's necessarily the stories themselves that grip me. It's the animation in his face and the way that he brings a story to life that makes me smile and connect.

Now, as his dementia progresses, there are gaps in his stories and words elude him in a way they didn't before. BUT his animated way of bringing a story to life has not changed one bit. His belly laugh and facial expressions are all as they have always been. The one thing that has changed is the way he's now brought his wife Cath into the fold. He has gone from a solo act to a double act, and he pulls it off perfectly. Cath is one of the most patient people I have ever met. Maybe it's the nurse in her, but there's also so much more to her. She exudes calmness without a spoken word and makes you feel safe and comforted.

She is now Michael's rock, and she provides that strength for him in a most dignified way that he takes and uses to his advantage. Michael knows that as he, in full animation mode, gets stuck on a word or a part of a story, he defaults to Cath. She in turn fills in the gaps (sometimes she takes a bit to catch the thread) and Michael cuts back in when he feels comfortable to resume the story.

Although he must feel incredibly frustrated on the inside, he trusts Cath enough to help him through the moments he needs her. But the story remains 100% his for the telling. I enjoy every moment of this, and it warms my heart to see what's possible when someone feels truly supported to be who they want to be.

Cath doesn't take over the whole story. She is purely the gap filler. And she does so with love and compassion. She gives the story back to its rightful owner. I look at Michael with intent and even when Cath is filling in the gaps, I still look at Michael for his reaction because I can see in his face he is still telling and living the story even when the words aren't his.

'Feeling supported allows me to be his wife and not his carer'.

-Wife of husband with dementia-

Research is telling us that …

Relationship-centred programs foster the building of relationship characteristics which include friendship, understanding of experience and development of trust. They leave clients and family members feeling valued and appreciated and have the potential to lead to positive dementia care experiences within community settings. Relationship-centred care isn't intended as a one-way relationship resulting in dependency. It's intended to create a relationship in which people may both give and receive care and feel valued from the experience.

Providing families with a seat at the table

Families are so well placed to make a difference in the life of someone with dementia but often lack the knowledge, training and resources, and the opportunity for their skills to be effectively utilised. With more robust education programs, families can more effectively learn about dementia and the associated care required, roles they might play and how they might support other service providers in their practice and determine how the future will unfold for them and their family member with dementia.

Family members can offer an untapped dimension to care but only when they're included in a teamwork model and their contributions valued. Together the team has the potential to achieve so much more than ever thought possible. By including families at the table, making them a part of the broader care team, friction that can sometimes sit between them and staff can be minimised. Stronger relationships can be formed with more opportunity to share in the achievements and wins associated with supporting someone with dementia that often go unnoticed.

Dear Family Member,

It's important for you to know we try to provide the best personal and clinical care we possibly can, but unfortunately dementia brings with it so many challenges and ultimately lets everyone down. We aren't trained in preparing you for what's to come. We're often not prepared ourselves which often leaves us feeling helpless and deflated. We dearly want to do more for you but often there isn't time. A shift for us is about getting all the jobs done, and the result is we miss the opportunity to connect with you and your loved one, to share in the day your family member is having, to sit for a moment and share in your visit.

There are always more important things that need to be done first, and as one shift draws to a close, the craziness of the next one starts all over again. We want to let you know that you're surrounded by staff with caring hearts who are so often feeling just as lost as you. As the end draws near for your family member we're often just as unprepared as you are.

We just aren't ready because we haven't been shown how. And when we say ready, we don't mean in terms of providing appropriate clinical and personal care, but in a way where we together can build an all-encompassing, supportive cocoon around everyone surrounding the person in the final stages of dementia. We too shed tears for the loss of your loved one, although they are tears that often go unseen.

We know that everyone needs to surround and strengthen connections around the person with dementia. We want to help build a community of connection and compassion to embrace all involved. What would be ideal is to be in a better position to involve families in a more tangible way, to assist us with the things we don't have time to do, things that you were doing just fine when your family member lived with you in the community. We'd love to hand you back the keys, to say it's your turn to drive again.

We acknowledge that you need more from us, and together we could explore new avenues for providing care that make a real difference. No one should be going it alone, and that includes you. You were the ones that were ready all along for us.

The system should have stepped up and been who you needed us to be. Unfortunately, we weren't ready and that reality hits us hard. We, as much as anyone, want things to change, so we can stand together with you and your family, to work together on new beginnings, to take the next steps together.

We aren't perfect but we care more than you can imagine and find ourselves on a learning curve like never before. Things are changing. We're finally beginning to better position ourselves for creating a new phase in dementia care where we learn from our failings from the past.

So many of us are committed to doing things differently and playing the role we've always wanted to play. We want to provide the service we thought we'd signed up for in the first place.

Together we can take dementia support to a whole new level and ensure that no one impacted by the advancing stages of dementia is ever alone again. It's your turn to drive again, to support us in our practice, and this time, we're coming along for the ride.

From Aged Care staff

When forces combine

There's no one in the world who knows what a family member is going through like the family member going through it, or someone that's gone through a similar experience. Families often have no choice but to just 'get on with it' and try to adjust to the ongoing pressures they face. Part of creating a united front for service providers is bringing families together to support each other and being more open to sharing in their lived experiences.

While it's beneficial to have the opportunity to offload feelings in a group setting, it's also a perfect opportunity to extend a group by empowering them to take ownership and control of what's to come, to set expectations and to define how such expectations could be met. When a group is able to work together to problem solve and come up with solutions, it becomes the driving force.

Providing opportunity for families to connect with each other is a unique type of support that can't be replicated in any other way. They have an ability to speak to another who, at that exact moment, understands exactly what they're going through, with no clarification needed. An opportunity is created to form a network from which strength can be created and bonds formed for facing the future of dementia care together rather than as a separate entity.

This shared journey helps to problem solve and navigate what is to come in a way that truly shares the load. Support groups are a fantastic starting point, but there's so much more we can do in this space to give families back a sense of control knowing they're not going it alone.

Finding one's people lightens a weight they alone should not carry.

-Wendy Hall-

Creating a local community of support

Putting dementia out in the public arena means so many more members of our communities can play their part in making a difference at a local level. Within Australia, around 70% of people with a diagnosis of dementia live within the community. That's a significant number who don't necessarily need any help on a given day but may find themselves at times needing to be pointed in the right direction.

In order to achieve this, dementia must no longer stay tucked away in the health and aged care world. Many living within communities want to be involved in supporting their neighbour with dementia. They want to support them and make a difference in their world, ensuring those who may be more vulnerable are assisted. The reality is they may hold back, decide not to get involved purely because they're not exactly sure what they should be doing.

Every now and then someone living independently with dementia goes missing. They take the dog for the same walk they've gone on for the last ten years and for some reason on a given day, they don't make it home. Emergency services ultimately become involved and search parties are formed.

What's interesting to note is it's often a concerned member of the public that crosses their path, who takes an interest in a media story about them and becomes a part of their reconnection with family. The more we educate and include our communities, the earlier someone may be identified as requiring assistance in any setting.

Dear Broader Community Member,

I want to provide you with an insight into what dementia looks like within your local community. You may think you haven't come across it before, but you have. Every day people living with dementia walk past you in the street, the shopping centre, hairdresser, and the doctor's surgery.

You may not recognise that they are living with dementia, but you may sense something's not quite right. How do you respond? By uncomfortably looking away, or do you offer a friendly smile? They may just continue on their way, like any of us just trying to blend into our surrounds, but sometimes there's a look in their eyes that can tell you they're not sure where they should be heading next.

When someone with dementia is out in public with a family member, family are often hoping things will all go smoothly, that the person will remain calm, that they won't be put in a situation where they respond in a way that may be regarded as anti-social, while trying to briskly get the person home to somewhere quieter, where everyone can collect their thoughts. Those living with dementia and their families need your support. You can play an important role in everyday life for those in the community impacted by dementia.

I'm asking for you to see the person for who they are and not for the person you see in a moment of chaos. If only you saw the struggles they face, the challenges they so desperately try to meet, the normality they try to create. They are attempting to blend into a world where it's so easy to stand out, to be different, to be judged, to be criticised.

But if you could see into their world, even just a snapshot into the hardships they face, you would not look away. You would do things differently and lend a hand. So please step forward and assist. Don't take over but offer support in such a way that leaves the person's dignity intact. Never underestimate the difference your smile might make to someone's day.

Thank you.
From a Dementia Doula

Catherine's story ...

Catherine was supporting her mum in a higher care home, and shared her experience after reading *Dementia can't take everything!* Her story provides a good example of what can be achieved by everyone coming together to work towards a common goal which results in a positive outcome for the person living with dementia, and less trauma for all involved.

Catherine's mother, Evelyn, had experienced what had been described as an 'episode' one evening. She became aggressive towards staff, throwing things and hitting out at them. She was also refusing to take her medications. Catherine was called and was informed about the events unfolding and told ambulance and police were on their way. Her first words to staff were, 'You are not sending her to hospital!'.

She knew that confusion could be a major issue for someone with dementia and taking them to hospital and into an unfamiliar environment was not going to help. Catherine was also conscious of what she felt was wasting ambulance resources. She told care home staff she was on her way.

Catherine arrived and worked with Paramedics to settle her mother and finally de-fused the situation. She praised the ambulance officers who were understanding and felt comfortable cancelling police.

Catherine returned to the care home the following morning to visit her mother, and as she referred to the chaos that had ensued the night before, her mother looked at her confused as to what she was talking about with no recall of events.

This story highlights that with simple interventions, the outcome changed from Catherine's mother being possibly sedated and restrained in a hospital setting to calmly waking in her own familiar environment and enjoying a quality visit from her daughter.

Preparing for a better tomorrow ...

What could you do to foster better communication ......?

Family perspective ...

'We don't want to take over, we just want to know what you need from us.'

- Daughter of dad with dementia –

Just remember that ...

When surrounding someone with dementia with a community of connection, it's like handing them back the keys.

-Wendy Hall-

8 • Preparing for a better day

'Very few interventions exist that try to enhance equal family-staff partnerships in nursing homes. Future interventions should pay specific attention to mutual exchange and reciprocity between family and staff.'

- Backhaus et. al., 2020 p.14

Imagine …

Imagine any given day having a plan attached to it rather than blindly trying to just survive it.

A better day for families is having a feeling of security, knowing Advanced Care Directives are completed and in place, and if not, being guided by someone like a Dementia Doula in the creation of one. A directive brought together and based on the person and their life story, without feeling pressured to get it perfect or right, helps families feel comfort in having made a start on their loved one's wishes. Peace can then be in knowing that all surrounding their loved one are doing everything possible to support, but not hasten, a peaceful and comfortable death within the final stage of dementia.

Preparing for a better day is planning for the future so families can come back to living for today. For this to be achieved, families must have the following in place:

- Opportunity for facilitated conversations earlier about advance care planning.

- Support and guidance measures in place that are clearly documented.

- A way to feel empowered in conversations with health and care providers.

- A plan for a seamless flow through community and residential sectors.

- A plan in place and an understanding of what is to come.

- An understanding of when palliative approach measures should be initiated and put in place.

When these areas are adequately covered, and families feel more comfortable in the role they play, the dementia care experience is enhanced for all involved. The flow-on effect from palliative approach options being discussed earlier with families is a marked decrease in the rate of unnecessary medical treatment that doesn't support comfort measures. Families and staff will also feel more comfortable in the support required by the person with dementia leading to a decrease in the rate of unnecessary hospital presentations.

Through the provision of regular and ongoing education sessions for families and staff, everyone involved can be on the same page with families better placed to support staff with end-of-life practices.

Family members who feel supported and enabled are better positioned for taking the initiative for improving care provision. They may also support staff in ensuring there is a more consistent approach to the timely application of palliative care practices.

The most important way to prepare for better days ahead is to ensure families are best equipped for answering the following questions:

1. What does care and support mean to you and your loved one?

2. What role do you play and/or want to play into the future?

3. What would you want from the aged care system moving forward?

4. What would future comfort care look like if you could paint the picture?

Honesty without judgement

Staff can't be everywhere all the time. Simple conversations can ensure that a dialogue is created, and families know who they can comfortably connect with should the need arise. The following points may assist families with starting a conversation with staff or management:

- Letting staff know of changes in the person with dementia that may only be subtle and easily overlooked.

- Passing on information to staff or management about issues that will likely require further investigation. For example, safety concerns.

- Asking for a formalised way to pass on feedback to be considered.

- Having the opportunity to have more input into a family member's care and what that might look like.

Dear Care Staff,

Firstly, I would like to sincerely say "thank you" for the support that you give to my husband, which in turn supports me. It can be a thankless job at times, but then also a very rewarding one, with special moments.

Can I please ask, that you always treat him with respect, dignity, compassion and understanding. You are going to need a lot of patience and tolerance. Allow him to continue to do whatever he is able to do, but at times with your help. Support him in having experiences that he really enjoys.

I hope that you have had some training in dementia care, as this is a specialised area of care in understanding specifically about dementia, and what can be confusing and difficult for a person living with dementia.

Learn everything that there is to know about the person that you are caring for, especially their likes and dislikes. Learn about their life. You can always learn more about dementia. Once again thank you for helping our family.

Family carer - Jenny

When enough never seems enough

As a Dementia Doula, I want families to know I expect nothing from them in any given moment. I never want them to feel like they need to make urgent decisions, (unless, of course, for a medical event). For me, preparing for tomorrow is about slowing down today. I often say to my clients that when they meet with service providers there's often an element of stress attached, decisions to be made, sometimes in haste, and information to be digested quickly.

This can mean little time left for answering the questions families forgot they wanted to ask in the first place. I make it clear to families that when they see me, I don't want them to feel stressed. I want them to feel like they can finally take a deep breath and have the opportunity to bring a perspective to what they're facing.

Often when someone is diagnosed with dementia there's the initial shock and sadness followed by a franticness to get things in place as soon as possible, to try and wade through a mountain of well-meaning brochures or put them straight onto the last pile they were given.

It all happens so fast and after things do start to settle, families commonly find themselves going it alone. But the questions still remain and often without anywhere to put them. Life begins to gain momentum and the crazy ride begins with families feeling like they just need to hold on for dear life.

Families often wish there was a pause button, an opportunity to take a moment, to try to work out whether there is any way to slow things down, put things in their rightful place so that every day doesn't start with a sigh. Questions flow like, 'Where do we start?', 'Where should we head next?', 'What are we supposed to do now?'. All these are valid questions that can't necessarily be answered in a glossy brochure when life has suddenly been turned upside down.

I remember sitting with a family around their dining room table with a daughter in tears because she didn't know what to do for her mother. As we talked through things they perhaps needed to consider putting in place, the daughter commented she'd already done everything suggested. It felt like life for her was on a loop.

Even though she'd already done so much and put so many things in place, she still couldn't allow herself a moment to take her foot off the pedal. The rest of our catch-up was about recognising and acknowledging the effort she'd already put in and how far ahead they already were as a family. As her mother with dementia joined us at the table, she too, expressed her appreciation of her daughter, which could only have happened by slowing everything down and validating her actions.

Getting back on course

Caring for someone with dementia 24 hours a day, 7 days a week, 365 days of the year is no mean feat. Most of us could never even begin to imagine how hard that must be and the toll it takes on a person.

What those surrounding a family member in this position need to consider is avoiding well-meaning advice that often falls short of its intended target. What we need is for families to help us to better understand their position and what they need from us on a regular basis.

Many of us are well intentioned when offering support but we need to remember there's a line to never cross. Family members in a direct care role get to steer the ship and the rest of us become the crew. The analogy is one I shared with a family who were struggling to work out the role each would play. Well-meaning family members, who commonly try to fix and manage and support those whom they feel need it, were encouraging a particular path the primary care giver didn't wish to take.

The primary carer was overwhelmed by everything going on around them and tired from being a fulltime carer. They felt they had no more to give and that a more supported care environment may be warranted. This moment in time is difficult enough as it is but often comes with convincing others that the decision being made is the right one.

When discussing where everyone in a family unit is positioned, I sometimes find it easier to discuss by putting the primary carer at the helm of the ship. They are the captain and it's ultimately their ship to steer. They call the shots. It's important to reassure a primary carer that they can override the suggestions of well-meaning others, that they may politely decline support that may not have even been asked for.

But while a primary carer is captain of the ship, they sometimes need reminding that they still need a crew behind them. The crew will support them when the seas get rough and the waves pound against the side of the ship. The reality is, with heightened emotions and without common ground, family members often go it alone with any clear direction.

What can happen is that a primary carer steers into unchartered waters with no true idea or understanding about where they're heading or what the final destination will be. They try to navigate the waters and do so without the right equipment or knowing what assistance they need to safely get there.

If the captain of the ship isn't informed or doesn't understand the role they play, they may find themselves looking back at the rest of the crew. The crew is desperately needed and awaiting further instruction and not knowing what to say. If they don't receive clear orders, they'll make it up too. They may just start throwing ropes and equipment around with no clear intention of where it will all land.

When the captain yells back at them to stop, to put the ropes down because they don't know what they're doing, that they aren't actually helping at all, that they aren't making the job any easier, it's often then that fractures begin to form.

The crew attempts to get the captain to make decisions about the course they think should be taken and the direction they should head. But the captain might just want to drift for a while, to try and take in what's happening and plot a new course to take.

Looking back at the crew, the captain may find themselves just shouting orders and instructions, telling everyone they don't understand the pressures they face. Often the crew are as directionless as the captain, with everyone feeling like they should at least be doing something.

If clear directions don't come, then others are just going to make it up anyway, because that's what happens when we love and care about the welfare of another person. We so desperately want to help and take away the pain and the burden that sometimes it's perceived that we're just trying to take over.

Dementia brings with it smooth and rough seas, sunny days, and stormy nights, all of which need a crew that is mostly on the same page to help navigate what's to come. There are so many unknowns with dementia, but at the same time there are so many certainties, and with this brings something to plan for. To create a contingency not during a crisis but for when a crisis hits. We don't want everyone preparing for what the storm will bring when the storm has already hit.

Nobody does their best work during this time and what happens is everyone involved becomes reactionary. They ad lib. They throw out the life buoys even if no one is drowning. We know the rough seas are coming, so today is the day to make that plan, to get everyone who wants to be involved to the table and ask them to listen, assure them that question time will come at the end, and they'll know exactly what's required of them.

By empowering a primary carer, they become better placed to inform others what they'll possibly need from them, not necessarily today, but when the time comes. All will hopefully fall into place without any need for asking. Because when those hard times hit, we don't want families having to ask or explain themselves; they'll just need others to know what their roles are and to assume them.

There'll be a community around them who will know their name is on the list and the role they will play. They will step up when it's needed most and answer the call to action. They can leave the primary carer to steer the ship while deciding on how and where they'll sail next.

This won't be a perfect science, but unless the conversation is started by someone, the conversation can go unheard when it's needed most. These unheard conversations can fracture families, not through lack of love or care, but because conversations can happen that are driven by emotion rather than by logic and practical thinking.

Putting things in their rightful place

Being organised is not just relevant to someone supporting a person living with dementia, but it is extremely useful during this time. There are times when we can feel overwhelmed, as if we're drowning, but when certain things are in place, the weight somehow seems to lighten. The following are things to consider in helping bring some structure to a family member's day:

1. Write down the 3 most important tasks for the day. Write them in a designated notepad or on a whiteboard. If they are the only things that get achieved, then there's at least a feeling of accomplishment. If they don't all get done, there's always tomorrow.

2. Create a 'to do list'. This again can be captured in a notebook that's referred to daily or maybe on an electronic device. The importance of this list is not in how long it gets but that it takes the pressure off someone having to remember. It frees up the mind for other things that may not be so cumbersome to remember.

3. Some 'to do lists' can sync with a mobile phone and be added to when things are remembered. A due date can then be included making everything even more streamlined.

4. If someone is out and about and thoughts pop into mind and their notebook isn't handy, a voice memo which is a feature of most mobile phones may suffice.

5. Do one thing at a time. While many people are great at multi-tasking, the added pressure this can place may eventually be the final straw for someone in a caring role. By doing one thing at a time there's better opportunity to get something finished rather than lots of things started.

6. Use the recycling bin or rubbish bin as much as possible rather than putting things away that 'may one day' be needed or useful.

7. Put in place a filing system containing red, yellow, blue and green folders. Things that 'must be done today' go into the green folder. Things that need to be actioned but not urgently into the yellow folder. Important contact information into the blue folder and appointments/referrals/prescriptions in the red one. It's important to find a simplified way to keep track of what's important on a day-to-day basis.

8. Learning to delegate is about feeling comfortable to ask others to assist with critical tasks in all areas of life. Something as simple as asking someone to take a family member to an appointment or picking up bread and milk on their way past a shop, may free up valuable and needed time for something else.

It takes a village

One of the biggest goals for us as Dementia Doulas is to bring together families in a way where they're better placed to support each other moving forward. When someone with dementia enters higher care, they instantly become part of a micro-community.

It's like a whole neighbourhood has been crammed into one location, all sharing space with others and connecting with people they wouldn't have otherwise met. Families enter this environment and are also transported into a community with other families who share a common and familiar story and yet are all unique too.

Ideally, we want to create a community within the community, empowering and enabling family members who may not be sure what they can and can't do, how they should behave and what's expected of them. If families are better connected right from the start, there's an opportunity to incorporate a type of buddy system where families take others under their wing and show them the way. They share in the unsettledness and are better placed in sharing strategies for what works or has worked for them and their family member with dementia.

This support can be reciprocated, and families instantly have a myriad of new names to add to their support network. I often highlight to families supporting someone in higher care that no one will know or understand what you're going through like the person you pass in the care home corridor. These impromptu meetings often result in casual greeting and conversation without any depth as to how each other might be feeling.

I think it's important to foster and build these relationships so that each can better support the other. Imagine a conversation that goes along the lines of, 'I'm going away on a short holiday and feel really bad I won't be able to pop in and see Dad. I'm worried he'll be upset until I get back'. To then hear another family member of another resident say, 'All good, I can pop in and see him if you like when I'm coming in to see Mum. I can bring in that magazine and those lollies you usually get him if you like. I do enjoy chatting with you dad when I visit Mum'. Care and support don't just have to come from the staff rostered on a given shift.

By giving family members a voice, they also have the potential to be a crucial part of any care team. It's often families that know why someone is calling out or what they're trying to say. Many will be reluctant to share what they think because they don't see the information they hold as being of any value.

It may be that the person they support is expressing concern about something that may have happened on the farm for many years and believe it's not relevant in today's context. But this information is important to care provision and may help staff understand why the person with dementia is so unsettled at certain times of the day.

Families will spend so much time with the person with dementia that they may pick up on subtle changes that need attention sooner rather than later, but often have no avenue through which to pass on such information. When subtle changes appear to a person's manner or disposition, family members may be left thinking staff are already across it or it probably isn't relevant. Empowering families to report and possibly even document the changes they note, they then become part of the solution.

Helen's story ...

I'm reminded of a story from Helen who had received a phone call at work advising that her teenage daughter had been rushed to hospital. Feeling panicked, she grabbed her bag and car keys and headed for the door while sharing why she had to leave in a such a hurry. I offered to take her to the hospital to make things smoother.

Without any other belongings Helen commenced the vigil by her daughter's side. While all went well, I called the next day to check in on Helen and she shared with me that she'd sat by her daughter's bed all night and was now out looking for coffee and breakfast, but the sticking point for her now was what she was wearing.

She'd asked her husband to bring in some things for them both and he'd packed a bag with things he thought she would need. This included the 'comfortable' change of clothing, Helen had requested. As well intentioned as he was, how was he to know what constituted 'comfortable' clothing? What he'd packed was what Helen referred to as 'her gardening clothes', those comfortable clothes you save for working outside because you're not fussed if they get damaged or dirty. They're not ones you'd ever wear out in public!

Now, the importance of this story is not in the well-meaning gesture of her husband, it was where it landed for her. Her husband wasn't to know how these clothes made her feel, and why would he? She had never have thought to tell him. It's important for all of us that we don't assume others know what our needs and wishes are. They're not mind readers, and unless we tell them, they'll never know.

This seemingly small issue made Helen feel self-conscious and uncomfortable walking around the city streets. This is an example of why conversations must be had early enough to capture not only the big things that are important but the small ones as well. At times, it's the little things that often have the greatest impact.

Highlighting this to families can assist them in considering what would happen to them if their voice was taken away tomorrow, and who would speak on their behalf. How well does someone close to them truly know them and be able to say what they will likely need or want? Just because someone is a life partner, friend, child, sibling or a parent, they don't know the intricacies of what make us tick and they won't know unless we tell them.

Preparing for a better tomorrow ...

What could you do to access more support ......?

Family perspective ...

'It's great to hear about what's going on, but this information would have been handier at the beginning. What I want to know now is what's to come, where's my mum heading?'

– Son of mother with dementia –

Just remember that ...

A lonely path always has room for one more.

-Wendy Hall-

9 • Creating moments that matter

'Although they often described disorientation and confusion, these memoir writers also demonstrated that they were still very much individuals with clearly differentiated identities.'

- Hernandez et. al., 2019, p.1167

Imagine ...

Imagine when families and staff learn to identify and celebrate the true wins in dementia care.

Experiences that bring joy should not just be reserved for the person with dementia but also contribute to meaningful opportunities for families as well. When achieving this balance where there's something in a connection for everyone, those moments are likely to happen more often and be more tailored to the person with dementia.

The importance of a coordinated approach to assisting families in preparation for creating connections can't be stressed enough. When more difficult conversations concerning advance care planning have been had earlier, the latter stages of dementia can then become a time where families can be encouraged to relax, take time to rest and just be in the moment, to better prepare for what's to come.

These previous conversations now become essential as they drive what the person with dementia wanted and how they hoped future care would unfold for them. Planning and creating moments that matter can often mean the difference between someone with dementia staying within their own comfortable surrounds with people they know or waking up in a hospital bed.

This may be the result if it was perceived nothing could be done to assist them in a time of distress. When planning is carried out for all facets of care early enough, care staff have more time to get on board and understand how things need to be rolled out in a timely manner.

Strategies for transitioning into higher care

When the time comes to consider higher care, being more purposeful in identifying and collecting things that bring comfort and connection to someone with dementia may also assist with the transition. The things that bring comfort to the person with dementia follow them in through the front door rather than being added to the list of losses experienced.

Helping someone with dementia to get settled into a new room, environment and routine may not be an easy or smooth process, but by better supporting them with objects that bring comfort or conversation, there's an opportunity to try to slow things down rather than try to keep up with the speed things so often seem to take.

The aged care sector is often a fast-paced environment with a lot of hurry up and wait and that's something we, as Dementia Doulas, assist families to take some sort of control over. Alongside strategies that support the person, it would be opportune to ask an aged care home what their transitioning into care program looks like and whether it lines up in any way with the one families are looking for.

One idea that may assist the person with dementia moving into higher care might be to visit a care environment well in advance of needing it, to become familiar with it, meet staff and other residents and to then go home again. Opportunity for this could be repeated over time so the final moving day isn't one fraught with stress and fear of the unknown.

Care environments that have a café or coffee shop onsite can prove useful for this very purpose and can assist someone with dementia in acclimatising and becoming familiar with new faces and the environment they'll find themselves residing in.

Families can also be involved and get a better feel for the environment and all staff working there over an extended period and at different times. This is something that can only be achieved if sufficient planning has been done in advance to ensure an adequate lead time.

The unfortunate reality is many families are pushed into making quick decisions with limited options available for meeting higher care needs. This is often based on a catastrophic event that forces their hand sooner than anticipated.

A letter from a mother to her son ...

Our son lived interstate and would fly home every 8 weeks to help me with my husband and give me a break.

Dear Ryan,

I would like to thank you for all your love, support, care and understanding that you gave to both Dad and I, during our experience of living with Younger Onset Dementia. Even though you lived interstate, I will never forget how every couple of months, you chose to come home to give me a break by caring for Dad yourself. It enabled me to have a break, recharge and then go back to caring for Dad when you went back home.

I will never forget the day, when you took Dad for a walk to McDonald's to get something to eat. There was a stranger watching from afar, and you left such an impression on her that she wrote you a message on a serviette and handed it to you.

She wrote, "Hey, my name is Steph. I was watching you before when I was driving. I just wanted you to know that to me you seem like an amazing person. I don't know if that's your father, grandfather, or a friend, but the way you are with them is perfect and it only took me 30 seconds to see what a beautiful person you are. There aren't many left like you. I hope you have a wonderful day and a brilliant life. Don't ever change. From Steph (a perfect stranger that you made smile)

I still have that serviette. Steph was so correct when she said you are an amazing, beautiful person. I will

never, ever forget what you did to support us both. Thank
you!!

All my love,
Mum xx (Jenny)

The thank yous that never come

When creating more moments that matter, we place a value on
the times that often go unnoticed, moments that become gifts
for those who do so much in supporting someone with
dementia. Dementia is an area where the spoken thank yous are
often few and far between. They're often hidden in the
traditional sense for how someone would commonly express
gratitude or appreciation for something someone else has said
or done. For someone living with dementia, thank you can be
physically impossible to say.

Although families don't necessarily support someone with
dementia expecting the thank yous in return, receiving one goes
a long way in acknowledging the commitment and the sacrifices
being made. Thank yous make any of us feel appreciated. Thank
yous validate the difference made to the life of another, that
what was done was noticed. When we reflect on a moment when
someone genuinely thanked us for something we'd done we
revel in the moment. It can elevate our mood. It can make us
want to do more and continue on.

Families deserve to be thanked. They need to feel heard and
appreciated for the sacrifices and the contributions they make,
for the betterment they bring to those they support living with
dementia. The subtle smiles, the look of peace and comfort or
the tapping of a hand are the hidden thank yous often missed.

These are subtle acknowledgements from the person with dementia. Moving forward in this space needs to be about creating more opportunities for the thank yous to be recognised and bottled up for families to remember and use later when times get tough.

In tribute to …

In loving memory of Judy (Mum). You made us laugh, laughed with us and loved us all fiercely until the end. Love you Mum, Karina xx

I would firstly like to thank the aged care and medical staff that cared for Mum for the kindness and compassion they showed Mum whilst she was in their care. My one wish would be that there was more intense training provided to carers and staff to provide them with the tools to provide the individual care required for dementia patients.

Mum had Lewy Body Dementia (Lewy Body), a form of dementia that goes hand in hand with Parkinson's Disease, which she was diagnosed with in her early 50s. Lewy Body took over my mum and turned her from a perfectly sane, kind, warm, caring, loving person into someone that we no longer recognised. She insisted that Dad was hiding drugs in the house, drug dealers were turning up at all times of the day and night to bash my brother (who no longer lived with Mum and Dad).

There were elephants outside in the back yard, mice crawling all over the floor and there was always a baby crying somewhere that needed rescuing. She also became aggressive, particularly towards Dad but me also. I lost count of the number of times she physically assaulted Dad or myself; we couldn't react, we just had to let her wear herself out. She would calm down and not remember any of it.

I often cry about that side of things; Mum without Lewy Body wouldn't have hurt a fly let alone assault family members. I know Mum got aggressive in the nursing home with both staff and other residents. I witnessed it and the staff also told me about things she had done. The staff were very understanding but the other residents weren't and that made my heart ache that they had to see her like that. A particular incident comes to mind when the staff couldn't calm Mum down and they called me to let me know (which happened often). By the time I got there, an ambulance had been called to take Mum to hospital for them 'to deal with her'. Mum had a resident bailed up in the dining room with staff trying to get her away from the situation. The more they tried, the angrier she got.

I liken it to dealing with a 2-year-old having a tantrum. Mum didn't recognise me at first, she was in such a state. I lowered my voice and reassured her that no one was trying to hurt her and that I needed her to go for a walk with me. It took a few minutes to convince her, but she did move away, and everyone breathed a sigh of relief. I understand the staff were scared and didn't know what to do, but sending Mum to hospital, a sterile environment that she didn't know, with staff she didn't know was not the answer and never would be. It would make things worse. Mum didn't need to be hospitalised, she didn't need to be medicated, she just needed understanding and someone to talk quietly to her and distract her with something to do (e.g., fold tea towels, read a magazine with someone).

Mum calmed down after sitting with me and having a coffee and a biscuit and a lovely chat about nothing. The paramedics had turned up by then, stood back and watched things unfold and thanked me for not insisting that they take her to hospital. They agreed, it is not the place for a dementia patient at all. So please, please don't send dementia patients to hospital or heavily medicate them because they are too hard to deal with. They aren't. They are just confused, scared little lambs that just need love, understanding, reassurance and someone to listen to them.

Karina

Sometimes the wins become hidden or overlooked during the chaos. In sharing Karina's story it's easy to miss the moment that mattered. She knew what made her mum react in certain ways and she played a pivotal role with staff and paramedics in assisting her mum to calm down and in turn alleviated the need for an unnecessary and traumatic hospital visit which would have likely resulted in her sedated and restrained, confused and frightened, trapped in a situation where she felt helpless and lost.

'Be thankful for your yesterdays because tomorrows may never be.'

-Wife of husband with dementia-

Creating togetherness

Moments that could result in a sense of happiness are often hidden under the layers of dementia in such a way that doesn't allow them to easily surface. Happiness is there for the taking or creating and it's important not to overthink how easily it can be achieved. I remember reading, *The little book of Hygge – The Danish way to live well*, an easy-to-read journal on the findings of happiness research.

Hygge isn't described as one specific thing. It is about living in the moment, a feeling of wellbeing, a quality of life generated from the simple things in life. The low to no cost things we often take for granted but have an invisible impact anyway. It's the 'ahhh', exhalation made after sitting down after a long day. It's the moment of joy when taking the first sip of a hot chocolate.

Hygge is the warm and textured rug you place over yourself as you sit by an open fire, watching the flames dancing without a care, listening to the logs crackling with the smell of a eucalyptus filled smoke wafting by. It can be the warm light streaming through a window on a cold winter's day.

These are the things that are important in life and give us permission to stop and be at one with our surrounds. These are the things that often get lost in the busyness of caring for someone with dementia and for someone trying to navigate life when living with dementia.

For me, hygge is a basketful of blankets on my lounge room floor, inviting anyone who feels a chill or just wanting something to wrap around their shoulders as they head outside. It's the candles both real and battery operated that add to a sense of peace and tranquility. It's the calming colours I choose to surround myself with.

And while I refer to hygge in the physical sense, these are images that can be created with the same effect within someone's mind when described by a family member. By knowing the person and what previously brought them joy, it becomes about recreating these moments in a more creative way. If a person with dementia enjoyed reading in a lounge chair by a window with a cup of tea, then the simple action of positioning a chair in an appropriate position with a lamp, knee rug and a book to hold can make a huge impact.

Even if reading has now become difficult, holding a book may bring back memories and the same pleasure. Ensure any props are okay to be damaged as the person may enjoy the feeling of the pages so much that they start tearing them out. Secondhand book shops are full of old books that could be utilised for this purpose. The tactile sensation created should be celebrated and not scolded, for it's a moment the person with dementia has chosen to enter and memories may be flowing for them.

The best part of hygge is its accessibility for everyone. While it provides ideas and benefits for supporting someone with dementia, there are also benefits for families, clinicians, and aged care staff. Hygge is something limited only by the imagination and doesn't need to cost a lot of money to be put in place effectively.

Sally's story ...

Sally was a volunteer working in a dementia specific unit in an aged care home and shared this story. While talking with a resident one day, she noticed Jack across the lounge area asleep in his chair. A man and his son appeared and stood beside Jack trying to wake him, 'Dad, Dad, Dad!' he kept saying, with no response from Jack. His son even tried lightly shaking his shoulder, but it appeared nothing was going to wake him from his slumber.

From across the way, another resident yelled, 'Just kick him!'. Jack's son just smiled, but instead he leant over and said, 'Merry Christmas for tomorrow, Dad, we'll catch up with you some other time', and with that, they left. Sally was concerned that Jack hadn't woken up and was about to move to check on him when she witnessed something she couldn't believe. Jack partially opened one eye and slowly turned his head to check if his son was still there.

What Sally realised was Jack had chosen not to interact with his son: a lesson that people with dementia can still pick up on whether connections are genuine in their delivery or awkward and uncomfortable. If we want moments to matter for someone with dementia, like anyone else, there must be sincerity when connecting with them, or it will have the potential to become another tick the box moment.

'I know I have a background in this area, but right now I just want to be a daughter.'

-Daughter of mother with dementia-

Preparing for a successful visit

Visiting someone with dementia can be difficult for families on many levels but can also be a time when memories can be shared and happiness experienced. What's needed for any successful visit is an understanding and realistic expectation for what the person with dementia can comprehend and contribute. Disappointment often ensues when the bar is set too high and the person with dementia fails to live up to the standard previously experienced.

When we, as Dementia Doulas, assist families in readjusting what a successful visit can look like, it opens the door for purposeful and meaningful engagement that's more about connection and moments being enjoyed by all. It's taking away the need to be right or recognised and focussing on what the person with dementia still has to give and stories that bring them joy.

These moments may need some consideration, an element of creativity, but being prepared for a visit takes pressure off families to feel like they need to perform or come up with inspiring dialogue on the spot. Families may use the opportunity to visit as a way to include other family members, friends or neighbours wanting to contribute.

They can encourage the writing of letters or cards, send along gift boxes or children's drawings, paintings or stories and poems they've written. All these simple prompts give families something to talk about and can be used to stimulate meaningful conversations. The responses from the person with dementia may leave families surprised at the connections that can still be made.

When visiting, timing is essential and shouldn't be about a commitment to a particular time on a specific day. Timing is also about self-evaluation of how a family member feels prior to a visit. If they are feeling flat or down, then a visit would be unadvisable. The person with dementia will pick up on these feelings and this may be detrimental to how they experience the visit. The same goes for the person with dementia. Should they be experiencing a day when they're not feeling their best due to something like lack of sleep or illness, a visit would again be better rescheduled to another time when both parties have the best of themselves to give the other.

Annette's story ...

Annette shared this story about a visit with her aunt living in higher supported care with advanced dementia. It had been some time since Annette had seen her aunt and she walked into her bedroom with little expectation. She knew time had lapsed since her last visit where she'd sat by her aunt's bedside while she dozed.

On this occasion, Annette was taken aback when her aunt's face lit up and she said, 'Oh, hello. It's been a while since I've seen you.' Annette was floored and couldn't believe her aunt was having what she could only think was a 'lucid' moment she'd often heard about.

She sat by her aunt's bedside, and they shared in the special recollections of times gone by, of family events and occasions and of places that brought back special memories. This was a time Annette could only ever have dreamt about and the hour flew by.

As Annette stood to leave, she took one last look at her aunt's happy expression and decided to use the bathroom on the way out. As she washed her hands, she looked in the mirror and a wave of realisation swept over her. She thought back to the visit and realised no names had been spoken, and in her reflection, she saw her own mother. The connection her aunt had thought she was having was with her own sister.

Names had not been important and in hindsight would have stifled the conversations that had flowed. Annette was filled with a happiness she found difficult to describe. She had gifted her aunt a moment with her own sister and she in return had experienced joy by sharing in moments that had once mattered to them both.

In tribute to …

In loving memory of Brian, a kind and caring man who was always willing to help others. From his loving wife, Anne

Reflections on the past:

One morning I got up a little after my husband to find him staring at the loose tea container which was full of water with him saying, 'Look at this - I don't know how that happened.' I responded, 'Well it couldn't have been me - I have only just walked in.' Seeing his look of confusion, I turned to the dog and asked if he had done it. This broke the ice and we proceeded to make tea with tea bags. Lesson from that was not to put the full packet of tea into the container.

Another day, I was offered a cup of coffee which I gratefully accepted. My husband took his with him down to his shed and after my first mouthful I decided to make my own, I discovered that he had put tea leaves into the jug, boiled it then poured that onto the coffee!

As I still worked part time, I received a call one day stating that he had got chops out for tea and was that alright. I then asked, 'What about the casserole that is in the fridge ready to heat up?'. Reply, 'Oh I fed that to the dogs.' Well, I didn't know whether to cry or laugh and did both but then decided that we had the best fed dogs in the neighbourhood! Interestingly when I got home, he had obviously thought about this and commented that it didn't have a name on it. Needless to say, after that everything in the fridge had names put on the dishes.

Watching TV quietly after he had gone to bed was a good way of winding down except when he decided to get up, go back, get up etc. His ritual was to say, 'Good night, God bless, I love you'. Each statement was followed by a kiss. After several interruptions one night I was getting really annoyed but then I decided it was better to be thankful for all the kisses I was getting.

There were other times when I was not as successful in coping, but I always tried to be patient as he had a been such a thoughtful man. I miss him still and always will.

Anne

Preparing for a better tomorrow ...

What could you do to assist with better connection ......?

Family perspective ...

'I wasn't going to come tonight; I was ready to give up on my dad. I just thought I couldn't deal with it anymore and my heart was broken. But now I have hope, I know there are things I can now do ...'

- Daughter of dad with dementia –

Just remember that ...

A Dementia Doula brings a calm to the chaos and a sense of hope within the moments thought lost.

-Wendy Hall-

10 • Putting families on the priority list

'Caregivers face many obstacles as they balance caregiving with other demands, including child rearing, career, and relationships. They are at increased risk for burden, stress, depression, and a variety of other health complications.'

Brodaty & Donkin, 2009, p.218

Imagine ...

Imagine when families have a self-care plan in place which is not just referred to when things are at breaking point but consulted as part of their daily ritual.

Self-care is a topic I've purposely put last because that is usually where, symbolically, family members and support providers place it. But my reasons for positioning it here are not the same. The hope is because it's the last thing that will be read, it will hopefully stick in the mind of those that need it most as an area of priority. The importance of this messaging is, if we don't look after families, and if they don't look after themselves, then it is the quality of life for the person with dementia they support that will ultimately suffer and they too will suffer. If that's not a driving force for all of us, then nothing will be.

I think of family members who, over the years have quietly and sadly shared with me, that they don't think they're doing enough, that they're letting everyone down, that they're lost and heartbroken. I take that moment, not dismissing concerns or offering positive affirmations, but instead opening up a discussion, with honesty and compassion, as to why they're feeling that way. Often by providing the opportunity for families to share their feelings gives them permission to talk and to simply be heard and they find their experience is validated.

The ultimate goal is to have families feel like they're leaving the dementia space in a better condition than how they found it. That future families stepping into the dementia realm will hopefully feel more comforted and supported than they did.

It's acknowledging what they went through wasn't for nothing, that they played a small role in making things better and were a valuable link in a never-ending chain. It's knowing the road their family member with dementia went along will pave a better way forward for others, that they didn't just end up a 'sufferer' or 'victim' but became a contributor, a pioneer, someone who was given a voice to educate us all in how it should be done.

The great journey of life … By Robbie

It began with cries and ended in tears.
It's the right time now, to look back at the years.
The good times, the bad, it was fun, it was sad.
Reflection of time and all that transpired.
Was once a gift that has now expired.
No turning back clocks or having regrets.

It's a lifetime of memories you never forget.

The journey of life begins, and it ends.
It's the life that was given, its paths and its bends.
Have no regrets with the life you once led.
Look only now to what lies ahead.
Those left behind in turmoil and grief.
Make the most of your lives for however brief.
As life is not given a guaranteed time.
Be thankful for your years as I was of mine …

It's ok not to be ok

You show up because you love. You show up because you care.
You show up with a broken heart. You show up in the
darkness. You always show up.

-Wendy Hall-

When caring for someone with dementia, families can fail to leave time for themselves. While feeling overwhelmed, exhausted and frustrated, trying to get through each day, they can feel like they're going from crisis to crisis or attempting to minimise disruptions. There's often an associated guilt experienced when attempting to take a well-deserved moment.

Families need to put themselves first, to create a sense of balance amongst the chaos of everyday life, to remove the guilt of self-care so they can feel calmer and more in control. The aim is to help to regain a better quality of life and enjoy special moments with those around them. It's reframing a mindset that ultimately benefits everyone involved, especially the person with dementia.

Dementia Doulas can assist families to know how to be nice to themselves, to try to alleviate any guilt that may be felt when it's time to have a day off, knowing that connection with someone with dementia isn't just about turning up every day, it's about genuine connection that's felt when someone feels in a good position to offer it.

Families don't give up because they no longer care but instead over frustrations of not being able to fix problems. They give up because their hearts continue to break over an extended period of time and they either can't bear the pain any longer, or they physically fall in a heap themselves.

But they never give up on caring. What they need is a scaffold around them, a community in place to provide support not for a day but for however long it takes, to prevent things from crumbling, to stop the ultimate fall.

Taking time for oneself is:

- Knowing the carer experience is an individual one, and no one can tell someone how they should feel.

- Taking time to navigate feelings and emotions that can leave a person surprised at what they're feeling and how they're responding to those around them.

- The importance of having someone trusted to express feelings to, and not being afraid to share emotions such as tears, anger, relief.

- Honouring the losses experienced through the writing of memories in a journal, writing letters, bringing together treasured precious possessions, planting a tree, writing a song.

- Preparing for difficult events that may trigger memories and sadness such as anniversaries, birthdays, reunions or when small reminders pop up.

- Taking one step at a time, knowing that there will likely be setbacks along the way, bringing back the focus to today.

- Taking care of physical health as the caring role can be exhausting. Incorporating a healthy diet and eating pattern, exercise and sleep will assist with the fuel the body needs to get through each day.

- Allowing time for a break to do things that are enjoyed, even if it might feel like it's all too hard.

- Trying relaxation or meditation to assist in managing stress and difficult emotions.

- Being clear about what would be helpful. Others will often not know how to help. So be clear in what's needed, even if it's someone to share thoughts with, assisting with feeding pets or perhaps helping with a few meals.

- Acknowledging that life feels overwhelming and consuming. An experienced health professional might assist with working through intense emotions and overcoming obstacles.

Easier said than done

What it comes back to is the importance of perspective. None of this is easy and families should never be encouraged to just 'get on with it'. Our role as Dementia Doulas is to assist families in feeling comfortable by not adding unnecessary weight to the burdens they already face; to help them to realise that they can't be everything to everybody, nor should they expect to be. The caring role needs to be about putting clear boundaries in place that remind someone when it's time to ask for help and they already know where that help can be found.

When families stray outside the boundaries of what they have to give, it waters down the parts that they're really good at that make a difference to the lives of the person with dementia they support, as well as to their own. When the bar for caring is raised too high, there's a risk that everyone will struggle. Boundaries keep all of us safe and protected from physical and emotional overload. By recognising boundaries, there's a chance to regain a quality of life, a sense of wellness and to enjoy precious moments with others.

In tribute to ...

In loving memory of Ralph, such a loving, kind, and caring family man. You fought so hard. Never to be forgotten, Jenny, Ryan, Melanie, and families.

Dear Ralph, (husband with dementia)

Through our experience with Dementia, you have taught me so many things, and I am a different person today as a result of this. I was taught to be patient and tolerant. I learnt to make the most of our time while we could, and to continue to do everything that you were still able to continue to do. To continue to live life to the fullest. You taught me to ask for help. You taught me to look after myself, so that I could continue to support you for as long as possible. As you were young and had to face so many obstacles due to this, I learnt how to fight for your rights, dignity and respect. I was taught strength, as whenever we had an obstacle, I always found a way around the challenge.

You taught me that you were always there, even if you may not have been able to communicate etc, and especially when others believed you could not recognise us anymore, we knew you were still there by the look on your face, the slight movement of your lips or the look in your eyes.

You taught me unconditional love, and as a result of this we ended up with many special experiences and memories.

Never ending love,
Jenny

Finding the joy

When living in a time of upheaval, families need to think about what brings them joy or assists with relaxation. They need to factor this in when going through the day-to-day motions of what needs doing, sifting through priorities. Prioritising things that bring joy can easily be pushed to the side. While there may be big things that bring joy such as going to the movies with a friend, it may also be in the little things like going out into the garden with a cup of tea, reading a chapter of a book, or watching a butterfly settle on a flower.

The things that bring joy need to be considered and captured. They must be consciously integrated into each day, so they don't fall by the way. They must be done regularly so they become habit forming. A self-care calendar might be useful, where things that bring joy and happiness are purposefully diarised. A self-care calendar gives family members permission to be in a moment carefully crafted just for them.

Allowing families this precious time and space acknowledges they don't have unlimited time to give. We want them to recognise the point when self-talk sets in and tries to convince them there is no time for them, that there's more important things they should be doing. The default should be to bring out the developed strategies such as a self-care calendar to aid as a buffer for when unhelpful dialogue enters someone's mind.

Kate's story ...

A few years ago, I spoke with Kate, a daughter whose mother had a diagnosis of dementia and lived at home with her father. Kate detailed the struggles her father faced as her mother's primary support and carer, while she, and her siblings, lived either overseas or interstate. She detailed the situation her family were facing and decisions that needed to be made. Kate talked of the need for extra care to support her mother in being able to stay at home in the community.

The issue was Kate's father was exhausted and completely overwhelmed; he had no more to give. He felt helpless and believed he could no longer provide the care Kate's mother needed. It was important for the family to come together to discuss what was next. The siblings believed that with further support, they could fulfill their mother's wish to stay within the family home. The guilt they felt in caring from afar, in not being there in the physical sense to assist their father in the way he needed, was also strong.

What was more important in this moment was for a conversation to occur, to become a united front and decide on a realistic and tangible way forward that took into account the needs of all involved. Often the biggest issue for families is not that they want to step away or shy away from the hard conversations, it's that they just don't know what it is they actually want or what they're asking for.

When families are given space to talk and be heard, to have the opportunity to tell their story and the anguish faced on a day-to-day basis, allowing them to share the struggles big or small that are real for them, there's often points identified along the way that provide insight into what the real issues are and a possible way forward.

When this opportunity for families is provided, they start to connect the dots, making decisions and bringing together a plan they believe will make a difference within their family unit for moving forward. Family discussions open up a way to get through it together, with practical solutions but also space to be honest about feelings and emotions being experienced.

Bringing in the cavalry

There are ways we can support this process and guide others to do the same. Within the family's community network there will likely be those who bring strength and can offer a sense of direction. These individuals can take up some slack and even coordinate others in being as involved as they wish to be. Support networks often move away not because they don't care but because they're not sure what to say or do. Including them in conversations allows them to take on roles as they feel able.

When guiding those that offer support to families on a day-to-day basis, whether they be friends, neighbours or work colleagues, the following may be useful in how to stay involved and connected:

- Encourage them to never be afraid to ask how the person is feeling, to understand that each day will be different for someone in a caring role and to take the time to listen and understand what they're going through.

- Continue talking about everyday life. The difficulties faced, and the losses experienced don't always need to be the topic of discussion.

- Asking families what they need and how they can offer help. Provide suggestions such as home cooked meals, doing the shopping, going for a walk or doing something enjoyable with them.

In tribute to ...

To my Big Brother,

It's hard to believe that you are no longer here on this earth – that I can't just pick up the phone and talk to you. The highlight of my week was to call and talk to you – sometimes I caught you on a less than good day and our conversations were short, but then there were so many more that were long and in such detail. They would be about when you were growing up and the stories about our grandparents I never got to meet, our brother who I really didn't get to know as he died far too early.

In the last years of your life, somehow the changes you experienced in your brain, made you softer and more emotionally connected when compared to the decades prior where the changes may have been the cause of responses so misunderstood by others, responses often at times taken exceptionally personally by those you loved the most.

Having heard the news of your sudden change in circumstances when you had fallen at home on Monday, to having a partial hip replacement on Tuesday, to the discovery of advanced cancer in your hip on Wednesday, to booking flights from Australia to the USA on Friday, to boarding the plane on the following Monday, it was all a blur at the time. There was never any question as to whether we would come to see you. Even in the middle of winter!

When we landed all jetlagged, we were taken straight to the hospital to see you. I will never forget the look on your face – it was as if I could see straight inside your heart – the gratitude, the love, the happiness. The fact that you didn't remember the whole picture as to why you were in hospital was insignificant compared to the love that filled that room. There were other family members there and, of course, once we are all together, it was the best feeling.

I had come prepared that there might be a funeral to attend – I had stayed up the night before we left on our journey searching for just the right photos – ones that I knew would be significant and tell some of your story.

I had no idea that we would have endless hours going through them together at your hospital bedside. Your doctor would ask if you knew who was in the room with you and of course you did. You even told her who was in the photos!

Only me and our sister were really aware that your days were not going to be as many as we all would have hoped. It was so very hard for your lovely wife of 54 years and your sons to accept that you were not going to be getting better in rehab for your hip.

You were so good to let us know you were in pain. It was just frustrating that those who looked after you would only ask you in the way they asked all their other patients who did not have dementia.

It was confusing for you to understand the context of the scale they used. The one where you rate your pain on a scale from 1-10. You responded 'not that bad' when in fact you were actually experiencing significant pain. I can't remember, but I believe that our sister was on to that quickly to insist that you had pain relief.

The push was to get you up and into rehab - to eat to get stronger when your body wasn't hungry and you didn't have the strength as you had begun to actively die. As the conversations turned to palliative care, it had only been 10 days since you fell.

No one really had time to adjust - we just kept going day by day. Your lovely wife made the decision to bring you home as she knew that is what you most wanted. You were still able to voice your desire.

I know that the next week was a time you were not always consciously aware of all that was around you - but I truly feel like you knew exactly who was there and that you were always surrounded by those who loved you dearly.

I hope you knew that we were all doing the best we could – our core team of the 5 of us (your wife, 2 sisters and husbands), your sons and their families were there with you as much as possible with your great grandchildren sweetly sitting next to your bedside, holding your hand. They were so young but they understood love. We had long nights where you would wake to speak and I would always tell you how handsome you were, and you laughed right up to the end.

Big brother, we tried our very best to take the best care of you. Often times we didn't know how but it was always in love and always with you at the centre. Three years on, you would be so pleased to know that your lovely wife is safe. She is taking care of herself and looks back at the decision to bring you home to die with fondest of memories amongst deep sorrow – in fact, we all do.

I want to thank you for teaching me so much about dying in such a short time – but that is what you did often in my life. We were 20 years difference in age, but in the end that gap was insignificant. I will always treasure the time we were able to spend together up to your last breath. I know you were aware of the love surrounding you and that it was so very hard to let go and transition to your death.

You were gracious to allow each of us to have private time with you, to say whatever we needed to say and to hold your hand that one last time. But we had to let you go as you'd been ready – your body had shut down. I love you and always will big brother. Thank you for allowing us to care for you and what we got in return was the most beautiful sense of closure, knowing we did all we could to live out your last days with dignity, love and significance.

With immense love & gratitude to you handsome,
Your little Sis

Preparing for a better tomorrow ...

What could you put in place today to better support yourself?

Family perspective ...

'Regret not the things that you did wrong but be thankful for all you got right.'

- Wife of husband with dementia –

Just remember that ...

You are admired more than you'll ever know as you quietly soldier on in the background, continuing to live a life of uncertainty.

-Wendy Hall-

Notes on Sources

1. Understanding the hand that's dealt

Brodaty, H. & Donkin, M. (2009), 'Family caregivers of people with dementia'. Dialogues in Clinical Neuroscience, vol. 11, No. 2, pp.217-228

Dementia Australia, (2022), 'Key facts and statistics', https://www.dementia.org.au/sites/default/files/2023-3/Prevalence-Data-2023-Facts-and-Stats.pdf

Alzheimer's Disease International – (2020), 'Dementia Statistics', https://www.alzint.org/about/dementia-facts-figures/dementia-statistics/

2. The reality of the day to day

Hernandez, E., Spencer, B., Faber, A. & Ewert, A. (2019), ''We are a Team'': Couple Identity and Memory Loss'. Dementia, vol. 18(3), pp1166-1180

3. Carrying the weight of dementia

Day, J.R., & Anderson, R.A. (2011), 'Review Article Compassion Fatigue: An Application of the Concept to Informal Caregivers of Family Members with Dementia', Nursing Research and Practice, vol. 2011, Article ID 408024, pp.1-10

Beyond Blue, (2022), 'Grief and Loss',
https://www.beyondblue.org.au/mental-health/grief-and-loss

Postle, E. '7 Warning Signs You Have Alzheimer's Spouse Grief'
https://www.griefandsympathy.com/alzheimer-spouse-grief.html

4. Planning for tomorrow

Stirling, C., McInerney, F., Andrews, S., Ashby, M., Toye, C., Donohue, C., Banks, S., & Robinson, A. (2014), 'A tool to aid talking about dementia and dying — Development and evaluation', PubMed, vol. 21(4), pp.337-343

5. Connections and reflections

Miron, A.M., Thompson, A.E., McFadden, S.H., & Ebert, A.R., (2019), 'Young Adults' Concerns and Coping Strategies Related to their Interactions with their Grandparents and Great-Grandparents with Dementia', Dementia, vol. 18(3) pp.1025–1041

Dementia Australia (2022), 'Tips for visiting',
https://www.dementia.org.au/sites/default/files/helpsheets/Helpsheet -TipsToAssistSocialEngagement02_TipsForVisiting_english.pdf

Dementia Australia (2022) 'Tips for caring from a distance', https://www.dementia.org.au/sites/default/files/helpsheets/Helpsheet TipsToAssistSocialEngagement06_TipsForCaringFromADistance_e nglish.pdf

6. Creative caring

Heath, P., Hughes, I., & Gosney, M.A. (2019), 'The validation of a memory box contents for patients with dementia', Age and Ageing, vol. 48(2), pp. 1–10

7. Navigating the path as a united front

Rosato, M., Leavey, G., Cooper, J., Cock, P., & Devine, P. (2019), 'Factors associated with public knowledge of and attitudes to dementia: A cross-sectional study', PLoS ONE 14(2), pp.1-13

Dementia Australia, (2022), 'Key facts and statistics', https://www.dementia.org.au/sites/default/files/2023-3/Prevalence-Data-2023-Facts-and-Stats.pdf

de Witt, L., & Fortune, D., (2019), 'Relationship-Centered Dementia Care: Insights from a Community-Based Culture Change Coalition', Dementia, vol. 18(3) 1146–1165

8. Preparing for a better day

Backhaus, R., Hoek, L.J.M., de Vries, E., van Haastregt, E.C.M., Hamers, J.P.H., & Verbeek Backhaus. H., (2020), 'Interventions to foster family inclusion in nursing homes for people with dementia: a systematic review', BMC Geriatrics, vol. 20:434, pp.1-17

Zen Habits, '27 Great Tips to Keep Your Life Organized', https://zenhabits.net/27-great-tips-to-keep-your-life-organized/

9. Creating moments that matter

Hernandez, E., Spencer, B., Faber, A. & Ewert, A. (2019), ''We are a Team'': Couple Identity and Memory Loss'. Dementia, vol. 18(3), pp1166-1180

Wiking, M., *The little book of hygge,* (Penguin Random House 2016) pg. 6

10. Putting families on the priority list

Brodaty, H. & Donkin, M. (2009), 'Family caregivers of people with dementia'. Dialogues in Clinical Neuroscience, vol. 11, No. 2, pp.217-228

Acknowledgments

Bringing, *Beyond the darkness of dementia* to life was such a privilege and I was excited by the enthusiasm that family members past and present showed in sharing their stories. All were happy for us to learn from their experiences and grow in our understanding of dementia care today and into the future. They bravely shared their stories to provide us with a glimpse into their lived experience of dementia. I know this inspiring act will empower others to do the same moving forward.

I would like to personally thank the following for their valuable contributions in making this book possible:

To Robbie, your unwavering belief in me is something I take forward every single day. Thank you for the opportunity to share this journey with you.

To Jenny, Sarah, Cath, Jenie, Karina, Monique, Anne, Lorrie and Ann-Marie, the biggest thank yous to you all. I am humbled by the trust you all placed in me to share your treasured stories. Stories that I acknowledge would not have been easy to write and ones that have stirred memories for some from long ago.

Please know you have all opened a door and paved the way for this to become a normal part of the dementia trajectory for families rather than something they must carry hidden inside.

A special mention and thank you to Rob and Doug. I came into the world of dementia 18 years ago thinking I knew all about dementia from my clinical past. I was quickly humbled when soon realising I knew nothing about dementia, what I brought was my intuitive and instinctive ability to connect.

You both graciously shared your knowledge and understanding of what it is to truly support families and those living with dementia. Your greatest teachings were to not just hear what families had to say but to listen to their stories, the words they chose to share, and to the often unspoken words.

To Nina and Lorrie, what would I do without your support? Your unwavering commitment to making tomorrow better for those impacted by advancing dementia will see us leave a legacy for others to continue to build on.

And finally, to my wonderful husband John and son Louis. You will never fully appreciate how much it means to have you by my side throughout everything I do. And to Mabel – my beautiful Dementia Doula Dog. When I see the joy you bring to those whose path you cross, you epitomise how to live and be in the moment and to appreciate the small things in life. To stop and smell the eucalyptus leaves and to make time to chat to those we pass on our walks.

Together we will make a difference.

Wendy Hall's library of dementia publications:

• Dementia can't take everything!

• The Dementia Doula

Each publication brings a different perspective for supporting those impacted by advancing dementia.

Available through:
www.dementiadoulas.com.au or online bookstores.

Part proceeds from sales benefits:
Community based programs ensuring families stay connected.